MALINGERY

Stealing The Truth

ABBEY STRAUSS

CONTENTS

Acknowledgments

Every project reflects the support of many. My thanks to colleagues who helped me discover and refine these ideas, to attorneys who let me assist in their work, and to all those who let me peek into their worlds. From these opportunities came a richer grasp of human behavior. Finally, a special thanks to David Yancor for the excellent editing and suggestions that so improved this project.

Dedication

Dedicated equally, and with profound appreciation, to all who have been either honest or dishonest with me.

Introduction

*\Ma*lin"ger*y \, n. The spirit or practices of a malingerer; malingering
MALINGER, to feign sickness (a falsehood)*

Truth is critical for the integrity and welfare of any community.

Proper decisions and sensible actions cannot be made if they rely on falsehoods. Behaviors that stem out of motivations to deceive in the name of a personal or political goal will ultimately destroy a community.

The rationalizations for lying generally fall into two camps. One camp is rooted in myriad religious, ethical and moral issues. This camp generally assumes the liar has unfettered free will.

The other camp bases their viewpoint on compelling research that supports the notion that certain groups of disease states facilitate mendacity (or permit prevarication). This camp observes that situations occur in which the decision-making process may not derive from an entirely free will. As such, it expands the reality and range of human behaviors in a confusing way because a medical condition—and not an issue of morality—could be the basis for some falsification.

For instance, a "lie" or a confabulation could emerge because of frontal lobe-based problems with executive planning. Consider a case of Pick's disease or dementia. These present with triads of poor concentration, poor recent memory and poor planning as a result of dorsolateral prefrontal degenerations.

These behavioral origins force us to re-consider the possibilities that behaviors which had historically been explained as evilness or wickedness should properly be explained as a possible medical aberration beyond the person's conscious control. What may have been easily labeled as an act of aberrant "free will" could very well be the opposite. Problematic choices may not be the product of evil, but of disease or some psychological devastation.

Perhaps all of the concepts of malingering, feigning, factitious disorders, self-serving political strategies, marketing, and outright lying, etc., might be better gathered and merged under a new umbrella of falsification disorders.

These core questions need to be asked about falsifications:

1. What makes a person feel the need to lie?
2. Is the lying more the product of willful deceit, or an altered mental status such as depression, psychosis, personality disorder or the difficulty in planning, as seen in dorsolateral or other executive system disorders?
3. Do those who falsify genuinely believe that the lie will not, or cannot, be exposed? How will they react if the falsification is discovered?

Behavior is the amalgam of biology and psychology. Free will proponents demand that we question how much free will and freedom we actually have in our choice-making processes.

Society must protect itself from falsifications. The mental health professional has a mandate to develop understandings that produce insights on how to civilly prevent falsifications.

Society must also be vigilant with respect to a "truth hawked as the truth" bias versus a fact. Every incident of potential malingering and every professional report starts as a heterodox,[1] which must be vigorously and objectively tested.

One ethical and pragmatic conundrum is the popular conceit that succeeding and surviving in our society often requires skills that use a degree of falsification. We all rationalize and sanction shades of falsifications in the name of achieving our own chosen goals. Our social dilemma is exacerbated when falsification strategies reinforce themselves when the goal is achieved through such means.

Malingering, or lying, is not a discrete event with firm boundaries. Malingering has dimensions. It is quite linear and therefore has shades of intensity and implication. We measure the intensity or implication of malingering according to the framework in which it exists. Psychologists seek testing strategies with which to identify and quantify malingering. The "continuum" aspects of malingering are ultimately mistakenly reported only in "binary" terms—that is, either "yes, it exists" or "no, it doesn't exist." A binary format means that everyone qualifies as a malingerer or not. For this reason, the best diagnostic format is analog because this gives us a continuum that allows both discrete endpoints as well as a middle.

Feigning memory impairment, often expressed as "I don't remember," or "I don't know," is not the same as malingering. The "absence" of a memory may be no more than a lie. Malingering, on the other hand, actually contains an abundance of "memory." Malingering is associated with the hope that the given information will be accepted as valid enough to persuade a person to act in a certain way or to excuse a person from some liability for a situation or action. Malingerers steal the truth from those who must make decisions based on a set of proffered and often false data.

Lying does not feign a condition—it merely proposes a false explanation for an event. Pure lying is motivated by the wish to change the nature of someone's association to an event. Traditional malingering wants to change the person's degree of responsibility for the event. Malingering uses lying just as a word processor uses a computer operating system.

My own impression of the literature on malingering and lying is that it focuses too narrowly on the detection of false arguments alone. The literature has the quality of wanting to act as the police detective who must protect us from the spoils of a lie. It has an "Ah-ha!—Gotcha!" quality.

The mental health professional has the scientific responsibility to drive past the gate of simple detection. Without biopsychosocial elaboration, an unadorned malingering diagnosis is insufficient in honest mental health circles, although it may be sufficient in the legal circles. Declaring someone a malingerer is as psychodynamically inadequate as when a physician says no more to a patient than "You have a fever." The base cause must be detected, but in looking more deeply into that cause, the findings may also reveal a moral coloring of the acts associated with the choice to malinger.

Paracelsus (1493–1541) preferred a chemical approach to medicine; this attraction still has many followers. Hippocratic thinking had a broader window—science would best advance by adding the physician's clinical observations of a disease to attempts to find the environmental cause for it. Combining these can then, hopefully, more accurately predict the course that the disease is likely to follow. The location of the cause allows for biopsychosocial influences.

Karl Menninger felt that, one day, crime could be considered, to a great extent, a symptom of a disease. Others discount such theories of the genesis of crime and insist that bad choices are deliberately made under the scope of a free personal will.

Section one of this book is the product of my personal observations, experiences and thoughts about malingering. I also propose, or in some cases, merely convey, the following types of malingering:

- traditional malingering,
- hierarchical malingering,
- iatrogenic malingering,
- malingering by proxy,
- malingered safety,
- malingered health and
- malingered superiority.

and these three styles of malingering:

- Offensive
- Defensive
- Psychotically or biologically based (which may be a confabulation)

CHAPTER ONE

Malingering Types

You can fool some of the people all of the time, and all of the people some of the time, but you can not fool all of the people all of the time. ~Abraham Lincoln~

'Types' – the proper representation of class of objects

Malingering is troublesome because we all do it. We develop a considerable set of skills and put substantial energy into demoting it from the ranks of psychopathy by calling it diplomacy, policy, or strategy. We also color, legitimize and rationalize it with our individual egocentrisms.

The term is also often used with the political expectation that merely suggesting malingering can incurably harm another person's reputation.[2] Lying can be a vile political tool:

"The broad mass of a nation…will more easily fall victim to a big lie than to a small one." Adolf Hitler, *Mein Kampf,* 1925

Malingering folds into the same notion as propaganda. Indeed, both words convey an association to dishonesty and lies. Consider one operational definition of propaganda:

"Propaganda consists of the planned use of any form of public or mass-produced communication designed to affect the minds and emotions of a given group for a specific purpose, whether military, economic, or political."[3]

The word "malingering" comes from an interesting source. As a verb, it means to exaggerate or feign illness in order to escape duty or work. The etymology suggests more illness than deceit since it is to "fake illnesses." The word originates from the French *malingre* which is to be "weak or sickly." It is also the basis of the word "malignant." The word also contains references to being corruptible or thin: *haingre* is to be "weak, thin," and *hager* is to be "thin or lean."[4] Also present is a connotation that the weakness is a cowardly weakness. Even the thesaurus in the Microsoft Word software program lists lazy, idle, slothful, apathetic, laid-back or lethargic as synonyms. Curiously, malingering is far from an idle or apathetic process—it is very active and industrious.

The word *histrionic* is related to malingering. The term stems from *histrio*, which is Latin for "actor." That which is "histrionic" is often dramatic or melodramatic. There is also usually a calculated script or plot which portrays an improbable or exaggerated state of affairs.

The word "oxymoron" also offers some insight into malingering. An oxymoron is the combination of incongruous words. Often these couplets are poetic plays on words and carry a truthful humor, a wisdom, or a political savvy. Commonly phrases as "lonely crowd" or "bittersweet" describe clever juxtapositions of complicated psychological states. Malingering is the combination of incongruous symptoms. Many view malingering as a foolish thing to do. Oxymoron comes from the root *oxy*, which means sharp or keen, and *moros*, which mean "foolish." An oxymoron captures the experiential paradox many of us experience in life. Some languages even have unique terms to convey the paradox of the opposites. The oxymoron user knows a real relationship exists between the two opposites. The malingerer knows that no real relationship exists between the two opposites.

Malingering can be divided into seven types and three styles. Each type is then further characterized by one or two of the three styles. These will be described below.

Types of malingering:
1. Standard, traditional malingering
2. Hierarchical malingering.
3. Malingered safety
4. Malingered health
5. Malingered superiority
6. Malingering by proxy

The three styles of malingering are:
1. Offensive
2. Defensive
3. Psychotically or biologically based (this may be a confabulation)

One of the endlessly perplexing, but intellectually stimulating aspects of the study of malingering is the challenge to identify a single theory of malingering. Most people are quite comfortable in describing the manifestations of malingering, but there is a viscous quandary when it comes to proposing a theory of malingering. Is malingering the product of mental disease, or is it the product of a nonstandard or ruthless free will? Can it be both? And why would someone choose an action contrary to the expected behavioral norms in a society?

Any theory of malingering has to grow out of and allow for the differing motivations for malingering. Malingering can also be considered a form of greed, but greed feeds the ego more than the body. Greed seeks more than is necessary for mere physical survival. One simple concept of malingering is that it is a survival technique.

Resnick proposed three subtypes of malingering: (1) Pure malingering—when there is total fabrication, (2) partial malingering—when some exaggeration of symptoms exist, and (3) false imputation—when the malingerer attributes his complaints to a situation that has little connection to the evolution of the symptoms.[5] These describe, but do not capture any core motivational differences, in contrast to the "styles" of malingering.

Rogers begins to address the motivations in his adaptational model of malingering.[6] He proposes that malingering has a business marketing plan flavor. The likelihood of malingering increases when the situation is adversarial, the personal stakes are high and there is a lack of practical substitute actions to resolve the problem. These better describe malingering than the Resnick system, but even Rogers fall short with respect to reaching into the core motivations for malingering.

Multiple motivations feed into the process behind any decision. People do not have the same range of available behaviors, tools and skills; many make decisions from only a restricted or even dysfunctional decision-making set of tools. A simple "snapshot" of a malingering act is not likely to accurately reflect either the complexity or the paucity of the processes leading up to the malingering.

Malingering can be closely associated to the two moral effects of shame or guilt. These will be further discussed elsewhere in the book. Inherent in the testing of malingering is a requirement to understand the person's ability to feel shame in response to an event. This inclination is, of course, tied to person's own comfort in lying to others as a method to reach a goal.[7]

Malingering is the desire to control. Sometimes the central motivation comes from arrogance. Sometimes fear is the impetus. Assuming or discovering that a patient is malingering frustrates the diagnostic process. The trying riddle lies within the mismatch of the "evidence" versus the "report" of a symptom. The challenge, however, is not to stop the diagnostic process once the nuisance or annoyance is felt. Unearthing suggestions of malingering ought to automatically proceed into at least two additional considerations: (1) perhaps the doctor's diagnostic skills are too limited to find the real pathology. What is thought to be faking may indeed be just an atypical or very subtle presentation of a real diagnosis. The nuisance felt by the doctor could very well stem from his own diagnostic limitations; (2) the clinical questioning needs to extend beyond the suspicion of malingering and into an exploration of what triggered the malingering act.

The legal system frequently excludes the malingered explanation for an act. Great caution against inaccuracies is demanded because of the implications to the defendant, victim and society. Defendants who feign illness to avoid penalty are malingerers. But a person who is insane cannot be held responsible for malingering. The McNaughton Rule[8] is commonly used as a test for insanity—the accused must not know the act was wrong.

Though malingering is most often seen as a feigning of illness, the opposite is also possible—someone may also feign health. For example, someone accused of sexual abuse may deny his pathology to avoid being added to a sexual predator list. Likewise, someone who denies the presence of hallucinations in order to be released from a hospital can also be considered as malingering health. It is not uncommon for extremely depressed people to say that they feel healthy enough to be released from hospitals in order to commit suicide. They lie to get their way.

To lie is to suggest something that is at "variance with the objective mind." This is a helpful concept to use with malingering: the proffered symptoms, conditions or history are at variance with the mind of the actor and the observer. However, the real variances may not be known when the symptoms are first presented. They will appear as the actor and the observer test, challenge, see the results of, and live with the tendered symptoms.

Traditional Malingering

The most common and banal presentation of malingering, which I call *traditional malingering*, follows a desire not to accept punishment or responsibility for some action. It can extend across scenarios that range from "I wasn't in my right mind…and should not be punished…" to "I am not the one who is ultimately responsible, and I should therefore not be fined for it…"

Malingering is also the diagnosis when someone feigns an illness to avoid going to a party or work. Those who falsely claim they were so sick they could not move their car before the parking meter expired are malingering.

Malingering does not necessarily mean that one denies having done something bad. The diagnostically pressing issues are to figure out the "cause" component of the "cause and effect" relationship. Consider a case of an assault—the defendant claims it happened but he was without any self-control. Or consider the events following an embezzlement—the embezzler admits he did it, but insisted he was in a manic state. Or finally consider a school teacher who called in sick and, as a result, the students missed an important class. In reality, though, the teacher wanted to spend time with his new girlfriend. If the assault was indeed without adequate behavioral self-control, the embezzler was actually not manic, or the teacher was indeed not sick, then all three malingered for personal gain.

At its heart, malingering is actually an act of circumventing responsibility or involvement. It is therefore an act of avoidance. The accused proposed that an unproven panic attack caused him to lose control of his automobile. He then had an accident. He claims no control over the events and no responsibility for the costly damages—the event was completely out of his control. The accused may be malingering.

Hierarchical Malingering

An equally common form can be called *hierarchical malingering*. The ultimate responsibility for an action is placed somewhere outside or away from the individual. The person contends he lacked the ability to "not act" in a way that caused harm. "I had no choice…"

The insurance claims adjustor whose ultimate goal is to save money for his company (a corporate gain motivation) seeks to deny benefits, which may cause a person to suffer. The adjuster will pass responsibility for the action onto a corporate policy with which he behaviorally aligned. The direct perpetrator of the harm claims no control over the decision-making process that caused harm. He blames someone else so he will not be held accountable. He believes his supervisor or the company itself should be punished.

And, then we have this type of situation —

"Yes, I was sick, but the reason was that that my Mom put bad food in my lunch box…it's not my fault I had to miss the test…"

This is *hierarchical malingering*, and it is a cloak we commonly use.

Malingered Safety

One of our social contracts is to be honest with each other. Nonetheless, we are often foot soldiers in the arena of competition. We accept grey areas of fraud-like deception to be acknowledged as business cleverness. How often does the applause go to the sales leader, despite his tactics and that he is not the purest and most ethical participant? Our society is profit-oriented and ethics often takes a back seat to sales results.

This is a real malingering variant—something is presented in such a fashion that the real substance is feigned. The hope is that the reaction to the tainted appearance will re-direct people to a specific goal. Obviously the "honest" social contract has widely-accepted loopholes.

For example, a corporation introduces a new medication. On the whole, it is safe, but some safety issues have been buried in the haste to market the product. The company may have determined that any financial loss caused by lawsuits related to safety flaws is statistically less daunting. However, some people do get sick. This corporate deception could be called "malingered safety," since the presentation is truly a designed and feigned overstatement of safety. This is especially true of compromised research studies, which are suddenly terminated and deep-sixed when results do not match positive corporate expectations. The public may be kept in the dark for years or decades.

Malingering can also be political even in regards to social or financial policy. The following is an example of malingering safety in regards to environmentally-induced illnesses:

Despite considerable scientific concern, the government insists that global warming is not as severe a threat as the majority of scientists contend. Therefore legislation is not passed to reduce greenhouse gases, and the government tells its populace that they are not in any danger. If this is done with the hope of maintaining the financial health of an industry, this is not merely a different interpretation of scientific data; this can be termed *"malingered safety."*

Malingering Health

Malingering health occurs when someone pretends to be healthier than they are. This would happen most often when someone wants to do something that they would not be allowed to do if they were sick. This type of malingering could also occur if someone was hiding an illness during a health insurance application or for a job. In a more nefarious form, it could also occur when one hides an infectious disease from a new sexual partner. Malingering health is often evident when psychiatric patients want to leave an inpatient unit, so they simply report that the hallucinations, depression, or whatever the major illness that brought him into the hospital in the first place, has been resolved. At times, malingering health can also be the product of denial about one's real condition.

Confabulation is similar to *malingering health* in that the symptoms are presented to give an impression. Confabulation is very commonly seen in the elderly. They want to appear better than they are, and in many cases their condition is an embarrassment to the confabulator.

When an elderly person with dementia is reported to "confabulate," it frequently follows an unusually traumatic personal event. It is clear that they want cover up their deficits—they know all too well their reality and the "confabulation fantasy" is actually a wish. Hirstein says that confabulation is the failure of normal checking and censoring—the confabulating person does not know that their answer is a fantasy and not reality. But when these elderly confabulators are questioned further, it is clear they usually know they are making up answers. It is not a confusion of fantasy or reality—it is a designed endeavor using what remaining cognitive skills they have to paint a certain picture about themselves. In more severe cases, however, such as a dense amnesia or an advanced dementia, the commitment to the obviously inaccurate answers usually stems from frontal lobe involvements or a psychosis. This is when there may no longer be any separation of reality and fantasy.

The word "confabulation" means to fill in the gaps. That assumes some conscious awareness of the gaps, which supports the common use of the term. The term "confabulation" is too ambiguous because it does not reflect the extent of cognitive impairment and the level of passionate commitment to the inaccuracies. Perhaps there should be "lesser" and "greater" forms of confabulation. The lesser form confabulator has more willful cognitive maneuvering, can be taught the truth about a situation, and is, therefore, closer to a malingering context. The greater form confabulator has less will-based maneuvering abilities and will not respond to guidance. This greater form does not know they are bridging memory gaps, so it is therefore suggestive of a more severe neurological impairment.

Confabulation can be considered a denial of illness. On the surface, lesser confabulation and malingering overlap. Any confabulator generally has problems organizing or integrating information, and so has to fill in gaps. In the lesser confabulator, some ego functioning remains that is sufficient to recognize that gaps exist. The malingerer has no problem organizing and integrating data and information. The lesser confabulator has both some level of neurological impairment in addition to some level of conscious motivation to deceive about oneself—there is a "ring of malingering" to it. The greater confabulator has no deceptive intent or awareness of deception—it is similar to a delirium. The world of the lesser confabulator, on the other hand, has some motivational component in the condition on display—it is a mixture of malingering and confabulation.

I have heard comments that confabulation is a form of lying or self-deception. However, self-deception and lying can only occur when the person knows the truth. A greater confabulator does not recognize the absurdity or irregular nature of his statements, even in the face of hard evidence. One who is malingering would always be able to separate true from false data, although it may be quite emotionally painful for them to do so. A person who is a pure malingerer, when confronted with contradictory information, might further develop a story to offset or integrate the contradictory information. People who only confabulate cannot do this.

Someone who is malingering ultimately acknowledges the falseness in their statements, but the greater confabulator genuinely believes their stories.

Can a confabulation actually be a delusion? A delusion might contribute to a confabulation, but a confabulation is generally tied to a medical event, which, if responsive to treatment, ought to then eliminate the confabulation. Delusions tend to last a much longer period of time and do not always respond to interventions. Delusions have a propensity to be more consistent across time and confabulations tend to be quickly forgotten.

Confabulation is often not associated with deliberate attempts to maliciously deceive and as such has been called "honest lying." "Confabulation" comes from the Latin *confabular,* which is itself a mixture of *con*, meaning "being together" and *fabulari,* which is "to speak." The verb is a variation of *fari* which later became "a fairy, or creatures known for their enchanting tales," hence, "to confabulate" is to converse casually, gab, enchant, and chatter. It is also defined as mixing fact with fiction, either unintentionally or intentionally. When a survey of definitions and insinuations are reviewed about the word, there are suggestions that it is not lying, in the purest sense, but it is in response (1) to an inability to recall the facts, (2) to normalize oneself or one's experiences for personal gain, (3) to shield or hide from the intolerable, (4) to idealize, or (5) to keep secrets.

Malingered Superiority

Malingered superiority is similar to malingered health. There are strong elements of fragile narcissism in this type, since it is often done to impress or win acceptance from others.

The nineteen-year-old felt shunned by the basketball team after he made repeated mistakes. So he left the team and drifted, over time, to a smaller group of equally disgruntled teenagers. He pretended through his stories to be much better at sports than he actually was. He would hide his real deficits by (1) insuring that he never played against someone who might beat him, or by (2) always offering excuses why he could not play, such as a sore ankle, fatigue or other obligations. He knew he must constantly guard against being forced to show the true limits of his skills.

Quite often, the search for the traditional "cause and effect relationship" ends up demanding a search for the "cause" of the "cause." Pretending to have superior skills or unique experiences to gain or maintain acceptance into a group is malingered superiority. The ego structures using falsifications to achieve this goal must be explored.

Iatrogenic Malingering

Pierre,[9] in 2003, suggested the term, "*iatrogenic malingering*." He reports that in his work with substance abusers, "many of these complaints represent mislabeled, embellished, or feigned symptoms that often rapidly abate within the protective milieu of the ward…" He continues, "rather than demonizing such complaints, we view them as a rational response to changes in the accessibility of psychiatric and social services to substance abusers…[and it is] the willful misrepresentation of symptoms in order to gain access to more comprehensive or higher-quality care." This raises the question of whether or not some who malingers in the criminal system may have chosen this method as a means of asking for help. This may in fact be a variant of the motivations seen in the "factitious disorder," except that in this case the disorder is not factitious.

Malingering by Proxy

Malingering by proxy has been discussed in a recent paper which reported a case of a thirteen-year-old whose parents instructed him to feign an immobile upper extremity for the purpose of winning a legal settlement.[10] That the child was taught by his parents to lie suggests tremendous sociopathy in the parents, and clearly the social models that this child may copy in life will be problematic. The child is growing up in a "halo effect" that supports feigning to achieve a goal.

Another variant of this is when someone dislikes an item, such as a radio or car. They do not want to keep it, but need an excuse to return or exchange it. There is some shame, embarrassment or inability to merely say, "I don't like it…" Instead, they fabricate stories, saying it is torn, or overheats, or is in some manner defective. This defect then creates the rationale for the return. Quite often there is nothing defective about the item, but a store will exchange it merely to keep the customer happy. Be that as it may, the owner's ethical sense may have allowed the person to malinger a problem with the item so they will not have to take the true responsibility of admitting that they simply did not like it.

The Kasdan article brings out another interesting point. "Pediatricians are often familiar with *factitious disorder by proxy*

(FDP), which manifests as a parent deceiving medical personnel by fabrication of injury or illness in his or her child. This diagnosis is often termed "Munchausen's syndrome by proxy." One criteria for FDP is that the motivation for the deception must be internal (i.e., emotional gain) rather than external (i.e., financial gain.)" The paper felt this was both malingering and FDP because of the goal of financial gain.

Elwyn and Ahmed[11] suggest that FDP behavior is far more prevalent than many people realize. They report that 9.3% of patients presenting with fevers of unknown origin are fictitious, that 2.6% of material presented by patients to be kidney stones were fraudulent, and that in Australia, 1.5% of infants brought to clinics as being "sick" were, in fact, cases of FDP. He points out that *patients* with a chronic factitious disorder tend to be unmarried men who are estranged from their families, but the *perpetrators* of factitious disorder tend to be mothers between the age of twenty and forty.

Factitious disorders have undoubtedly existed throughout history. In 1951, Asher noted that some patients went from medical organization to medical organization, asking to get treatment for feigned symptoms. This pattern was labeled as the Munchausen's syndrome after Baron von Munchhausen, a 17th century German Calvary officer. The Munchhausen syndrome is characterized by numerous abdominal surgical scars, an evasive manner, dramatic medical histories with uncertain clinical proof, and efforts to conceal clinical documents and history. Munchhausen syndrome has fallen into a subtype of factitious disorder. Currently, the diagnostic criteria for factitious disorder is the intentional feigning of signs and symptoms suggestive of a genuine illness, a motivation to assume the sick role, and the absence of external motivations for the behavior. If there is an external motivation, then it more properly falls into the category of malingering. Factitious disorder by proxy is when one person intentionally produces or feigns symptoms of an illness in another person who is under that individual's care, e.g., the care-giving daughter of an elderly parent. The psychodynamic etiologies of such behaviors are usually complex and covert. The etiologies can range from depression, narcissism, psychoses, or other motivations.

One of the great diagnostic challenges is to separate factitious disorder from multiple other somatoform disorders, such as conversion reactions, pain disorders that are psychologically based, somatization processes, dysmorphic disorders, or hypochondriasis. In the course of a clinical proposition, the suspected perpetrator may try to manipulate the diagnostic team. This may produce a foul response against those who challenge the perpetrators claims. By contrast, the doctors may receive praise and accolades from the patients if they are sympathetic to the claims. This speaks to the common problems when dealing with people with personality disorders and mixtures of sociopathy and narcissism.

There are real differences between a factitious disorder and malingering. Although both present with false symptoms, the factitious disordered person is usually looking for treatment. The malingerer is looking to avoid responsibility or an association with an event. Interestingly, I have seen malingerers back away from their malingering when treatment is proposed or actually initiated. Factitious disorders can occasionally co-exist with malingering in a complex weave of motivations.

A sixteen-year-old spoke to his mother about his growing and deepening depression. She was sufficiently concerned that she brought him to a psychiatrist. The young man was quite clever and well-read, so he reported many symptoms that are found in legitimate depressions. The psychiatrist and mother later agreed that an antidepressant trial was initially indicated, to be followed by psychotherapy. One week after beginning medications, the young man began to experience side-effects to the medicines. Although it was difficult for him, it was nonetheless very cathartic as well, because he admitted that his depression was a ruse to keep him out of school until a girl, who he had a crush on, moved away. He lied about the symptoms, but the pain of the treatment was worse than his need to malinger.

It is critical, therefore, to be as objectively accurate as possible when testing for malingering. This will be examined in much greater detail below, but some preliminary comments first. I have often wondered if some psychological testers, who find malingering so often, do so because of their own penchants and inclinations to malinger in their own lives. Is it that they emotionally identify and resonate with the test subject's psychological process, and so recognize from personal experience the mindset of a malingerer? Or do they project their own established proclivity to malinger into the person being tested? Is the finding of malingering actually a projection of how they would act if placed in a similar situation?

By contrast, those who find malingering less frequently may not have personally experienced the psychological need to malinger. It is a mistaken belief to assume that ample objectivity in the ego structures of all those testing, or of the accuracy of the testing instruments they use, exists among the mental health testing community. This is a massive problem and it brings a real bias to the testing community.

All testing must itself be checked against the framework in which the test was designed. Any test's accuracy is further defined by the standardizing population on which it is based. Every test is further limited and circumscribed by the *gestalt* and the finesse with which it is administered and graded. One such cautionary is the notion of the "Halo Effect."

The halo effect speaks to the demeanor of any relationship. It can be hostile, rigid, non-threatening, slow-paced, meticulous, mechanical, friendly, energetic, sleepy, or any other emotional or environmental characteristic which defines a relationship. If an examiner is predisposed to being cold or short-tempered, then that characteristic becomes the "halo" in which the testing or interview occurs. The use, awareness of, and presence of the halo effect is a critical variable in any relationship, but most specifically in psychiatric or psychological ones. The examiner must be aware of various motivational biases on both his and the patient's part. This may also include issues of transference and countertransferences. These biases can produce errors in any diagnostic evaluation.[12] It would require considerable mastery on the patient's part to maintain consistency of lying across many examiners, and if one examiner finds no malingering, and another does, then the differences may be found in either the presentation of the data or in the interpretation of the data. How the patient responds to the testing may reflect attitudes or other milieu or stylistic favoritisms—real or suspected— that the patient feels exists in the examiner. This is the halo effect.

In the late 1920's, the Western Electric Company did an experiment at their Hawthorne Plant to examine the effect of physical and environmental influences on the workplace. The result has been called the Hawthorne effect, which essentially says that an increase in worker productivity follows the psychological feeling of being made to feel important.

Initial improvement in a process of production caused by the obtrusive observation of that process. The effect was first noticed in the Hawthorne plant of Western Electric. Production increased not as a consequence of actual changes in working conditions introduced by the plant's management but because management demonstrated interest in such improvements. — Krippendorff[13,14]

The obvious extension of the Halo and Hawthorne effects is that the manner in which people react to a task is heavily persuaded by how they are treated when they are doing the task.

Adelman and Howard in 1984[15] note that the mere presence of a malingering allegation can grow into a pejorative implication which discredits the accused.[16] If the subject knows he is being evaluated as a possible malingerer, then the milieu is not favorable to a trustworthy evaluation until the examiner and the subject are able to develop an honest and trusting relationship.

A non-malingering patient who has been classified as malingering is often denied mental health care. Unfortunately, the most common tests for malingering are based on psychological pen and pencil tests and limited observations. Rarely does the diagnosis evolve from efforts to develop a bank of rich data that follow from substantial and sophisticated treatment trials. In truth, the malingering diagnosis, with its potential criminal manifestations and ramifications, is often based more on superficial clusters of symptoms than on deeply etiologic and treatment-associated investigations.

If a "truth" of malingering cannot be produced, than a "probability" is often offered. But every probability is plagued with both possible accuracies and inaccuracies. Any diagnosis taken from such a "probability" exists closer to rhetoric than fact:

Socrates said: *The fact is, as we said at the beginning of our discussion, that the aspiring speaker needs no knowledge of the truth about what is right or good...In courts of justice no attention is paid whatever to the truth about such topics; all that matters is plausibility...There are even some occasions when both prosecution and defense should positively suppress the facts in favor of probability, if the facts are improbable. Never mind the truth—pursue probability through thick and thin in every kind of speech; the whole secret of the art of speaking lies in consistent adherence to this principle.*

Phaedrus replied: *That is what those who claim to be professional teachers of rhetoric actually say, Socrates.* — Plato

Even in legally based cases, any data obtained from the tests and investigations should become the foundation of a treatment plan to audition the conclusions. But the legal system frequently lacks adequate time, financial resources, or access to get sophisticated psychiatric investigations and treatments in order to deal with causes of and offer treatment for possible malingering. Therefore, the need for simpler, more routine, and more reliable assessments of malingering warrants considerable study. The fear, however, is that these simple assessments, regardless of their statistical analyses of symptoms, will not capture the core psychological motivations for symptom feigning. Too often an accepted diagnosis is based more on probability, oratory and a rhetorical *lingua franca*.

This raises basic questions of diagnostic accuracy. Indeed, Kraepelin in 1920, said: *No experienced psychiatrist will deny there is an alarmingly large number of cases in which it seems impossible, in spite of the most careful observation, to make a firm diagnosis…it is becoming increasingly clear that we cannot distinguish satisfactorily between these two illnesses and this brings home the suspicion that our formulation of the problem may be incorrect.*[17] Inaccuracies stem from insufficient or biased observations and/or knowledge of the elemental events and processes that precede the pathology causing a diagnosis.

One confidence building element in testing for malingering would be to expose the "malingering symptoms" to active treatment and observe for positive responses and changes, as well as to measure the willingness to put up with the inconveniences or side effects of the treatment. Too often after a malingering diagnosis is suggested, there is no follow-up hard test to prove or falsify the diagnoses. It is expensive to test with treatments, so being able to reach a diagnosis without such testing is desired. The actual testing with treatment is the equivalent of a biopsy, rather than just palpating a lump.

The problem with the factitious disorders is that they may cascade into a set of new medical problems subsequent to the original intervention. So if someone had abdominal surgery on what was eventually learned to be a factitious disorder, then post-surgical complications, such as adhesions, may fuel further medical interventions that are in part factitious and in part iatrogenic. The interplay between these two processes can become incredibly complex and even self-perpetuating.

Devices validating the existence of any falsification disorder need to be so unbiased and immune from influence that any tester could not skew the results. All tests are inherently biased because they choose limited areas to question. It would be impossible to test every aspect of human motivation and behavior. Tests are designed with the hope that their selected questions touch on the correct core issues which can then give a precise diagnostic summary.

In reality, though, a test is merely suggestive of a diagnosis. If tests were so reliable, then only one test would be needed and no two examiners could arrive at different results. Tests routinely do not list the areas they do not explore, yet within these untested areas may be diagnostically critical material. In an ironic manner, a malingerer wants a conclusion based on incomplete data sets, and fortunately tests or testers often allow that to happen. The reasons a highly respected test produces conflicting results may lie more with the different testers than the tested.

A twenty-four-year-old man was arrested for robbing a store. He claimed he was told to do so by hallucinations that threatened and commanded. His reported symptoms were very suggestive of malingering. He was overheard telling another inmate that he was glad the court-appointed doctor only spent twenty minutes with him "...cause he didn't ask a lot of other questions...and I just said no to those questions he asked me."

A sophisticated interviewer will do more than objective testing. The interviewer wants the patient to elaborate on their own emotional states. Throughout the interview, there should be reflections back and forth to earlier statements and comments. These responses will layer themselves into consistent and inconsistent symptom clusters. The openness of a psychodynamic formatted interview also allows for cultural and other background material to be blended into the diagnostic formula.

The lack of definite data does not direct against a legitimate diagnosis.

A man was applying for disability, secondary to inexplicable chronic fatigue. The insurance company denied the claim. Subsequently, in court, the man's lawyer asked a physician, acting as an expert witness, how many diseases can exist in humans. The doctor estimated that there are probably several thousand possible diseases. The lawyer then astutely asked if people can have diseases about which we do not yet have any knowledge. The doctor said yes. The lawyer continued by asking if some clusters of symptoms might exist, but in fact the true etiology is still unknown to science. The doctor again said yes. The lawyer closed his questioning by asking the doctor if it was possible that his client's symptoms were legitimate, but that medical science could not yet explain why. The doctor agreed. The disability was granted.

Tests are also easily fooled. Tests measure how the person responds to the test. A test is a measure of the cognitive responses to questions. Test designers hope to produce tests that are more clever than the client's ability to see the pattern of questions. Tests for malingering are based on the perverse hope that the person will be honest with the testing questions. A central question is—why would someone be willing to lie about the symptoms, but be honest on the test?

Labeling someone as a malingerer, solely based on a printed test can be an uncorroborated and dangerous diagnostic practice. Test results cannot be assumed to have more truth than they actually have. Results merely gather symptoms associated with malingering, and therefore only offer a statistical projection to proffer a risk of malingering. These tests commonly do not explore the ego structure causing the malingering-like behaviors.

When a patient expects the examiner to believe his symptoms, yet the examiner finds that these symptoms violate natural regularities associated with the symptoms, it is as if a patient is requiring that the doctor accept pseudoscience.

For example, those who report parapsychological experiences may present strong evidence which, in their opinion, supports that these events really happened. The scientific knowledge, however, tells us that it did not. The examiner might initially accept this as good evidence that the reported symptoms or events are feigned, but this can be too simplistic. An unusual report should at least alert the examiner to consider the possibility of a new variation to a disease state. Also, the report might be the product of a religious belief. Disagreeing with a patient's report of the real presence of their symptoms does not remove the possibility that they are genuine to them. Malingering, though, is not genuine—even to the patients.

If and how a suspected malingerer believes in religious miracles and/or experiences has to be part of the diagnostic workup. There are three elements to consider in such an analysis: the style of the report or testimony itself, the nature of the unusual phenomena (i.e., roots, voodoo, miracles), and the application of natural or contemporary scientific law. In 1748, David Hume addressed these very issues[18] regarding how we should react when we are told that an unusual event has occurred.

A wise person must proportion his belief to the evidence. To do so, the person must consider how likely it is that the event would actually happen. This requires relying on our past experiences and knowledge that teaches us what type of acts can be seen in a particular set of circumstances.

Understanding why an event happens determines how liable the person is for the consequence of an event. The legal system separates the *responsibility* from the *motivation* for an act. Strict liability is the only consideration when the jury must decide if a defendant has committed a particular act. If the jury finds that he did commit the act, they are obligated to find the person guilty. But if the defendant was insane or suffered other uncontrollable burdens at the time of the act are separate issues from the question of whether the act was committed or not. The concept of *mens rea* proposes that the defendant's behavior must be willful and knowingly in violation of the social order. If a socially unacceptable act occurs, it begs the question: was the unacceptable behavior a predictable behavior of the defendant? Therefore, the ultimate legal and clinical issue to be explained is the intent of the act and the development of some sound understanding of the mitigators which led the person to act in an unacceptable manner. If the person has no control over the mitigators, then an insanity plea may be proper. If there is complete control over the mitigators, then a strict finding of complete responsibility would be the most appropriate conclusion.

Critics of the strict liability argument assert that punishment should not be imposed *holus-bolus* without consideration of the defendant's intention. These same critics like to appeal to the notion of some rehabilitative aspects of a punishment. This is done with the hope that rehabilitation will modify those mitigators in the defendant's mind that led to the unacceptable behavior. In actuality, mere incarceration does very little to re-form the mindset which led to the crime.

If the strict liability proponents had their way, then people who act in socially unacceptable ways must be branded as criminals.

This process removes the real-life dimensions of the defendant's mental state at the time of the crime. Supporters of the strict liability notion often claim that the fear of strict liability is a deterrent against proscribed behaviors. The record seems not to bear this out.

Fortunately, many courts separate the guilt phase of a trial—which looks to impose a liability for an act—and a penalty phase, which tries to bring to court some measure of the person's pre-criminal life so that any punishment reflects a proper combination of the legal requirements for punishment with the etiology and mitigators. It is often within the penalty phase that malingering can occur. This malingering can be packaged in the attorney's presentation of their arguments, or in the defendant's explanation of his motivations for the crime.

However, the motivations for malingering can be very different, and, as will be discussed below, it can be conceptualized as a process of either *offensive or defensive malingering*. These two malingering styles can reflect and separate the person's character make-up in a very remarkable way. But it is first necessary to examine the *mens rea* concept more thoroughly.

The *mens rea* concept states that the person knows he is doing something which he ought not to be doing. The concept rests on the premise that a person would not be behaviorally deterred if he lacks the mental ability to know that his action will violate the law. Most people understand what behaviors society accepts and does not accept, so a defense based on a lack of such knowledge would be extremely difficult to argue. Ignorance of the law rarely succeeds as a defense.

What deterrents against socially unwelcome behavior exist when the mental capacities are highly dysfunctional? Is there an essential mental element which is malfunctioning? Does this move a person into illegal behavior? Is this lack of self-deterrence the product of a mental, social or moral defect? These are some of the core challenges when trying to identify malingering.

The guilt phase of many trials looks at the strict liability issues. The penalty phase thereafter looks at the *gestalt* surrounding the illegal behaviors. However, if substantial evidence exists, the psychological gestalt can be brought into the guilt phase of a trial with the hope of winning a "not guilty by reason of insanity verdict."[19] This is based on the understanding that someone is not as guilty if they acted or caused injury through a pure accident or involuntary disease. To punish people for these conditions would outrage a community and would nullify the social expectations of the legal process. It would bring the justice system into disrepute. A legal system rigidly dealing with a policy of unyielding strict liability could itself become a menace to society.

Interestingly, those who malinger actually stabilize our system against overzealous strict liability. Dramatically, they force a deliberation of the mental elements beneath behaviors. A malingerer is more likely to design his symptoms in response to his perception of the "strict liability" issues that he faces. The offensive malingerer approaches it in a more calculated, annoyed, inconvenienced, businesslike and sociopathic style, while the defensive malingerer approaches the issues out of fear.

Understanding why malingering ultimately fails can be found in the core of some essential Darwinian concepts. The malingerer presents his data as if it was real. To be real is to be tangible, incarnate, and similarly experienced by other people in similar situations. Those who malinger are fighting for their safety and survival. They are hoping that they—through their malingering—will guarantee or enhance their survival. But unlike the natural selection seen in herds, in which some new behavior is genuinely suited to improved survivability, the malingerer is trying to force a natural selection based on a single individual's needs. And that need is inconsistent with the growth of communities. It is a natural selection battle between "me," and "we." Unless the "me" matches the need of the "we," the evolutionary line will die. With malingering, the "me" survival does not contribute to the "we" survival. Too often, any reference to Darwin is prematurely limited to biological evolution, but, in fact, it applies to social evolution as well. Quite obviously, aspects of our psyche feel the need for self-protection and self-perpetuation, and lying is a selfish evolutionary strategy. The mental health question is, "why can't the person survive by telling the truth?"

Malingering is a human-to-human interaction. People do not malinger in front of a deity when they are in need of help. This is because of the powerful belief that deities can look into our minds in ways that humans cannot. I often ask suspected malingerers if they are religious, and if so, what would God think of their illnesses.

That one's mind might be readable opens a fascinating motivational door. In all cases, a psychological examiner wants to measure something. Both types of malingerers reveal only that which is questioned or that which he chooses to reveal in the name of a goal. But the offensive malingerer blocks any emotional resonance with the examiner. The defensive malingerer wants resonance. The offensive malinger says, "no need to get closer, just accept what I tell you!" The defensive malingerer says, "Please—get closer and understand me."

We test the safety of emotional connections in part by a sense of emotional resonance. We experience this resonance as emotions. If the examiner rejects efforts to resonate with the patient, the patient reacts to the coolness—which may actually increase the chance of a false-positive report. Dealing with an invitation to resonate requires two elements—the examiner has to:

(a) be able to generate from within himself a sense that emotional resonance is accepted, and

(b) he has to make time to explore the psychological undressing that occurs when people begin to resonate and desire to be understood by someone else.

Elsewhere is a detailed discussion of why examiners differ in their findings. One factor is that the chosen test instruments (the examiner's own psyche is one of the instruments) cannot or will not capture the person's resonating inner self. This may be part of mirror neuron activities. This neurological system is hypothesized to be at least one basis for empathy and understanding.

Malingerers do not earn the label of the illnesses they stage because they do not suffer the truths of these illness. Instead, they steal the style of the illness for their own purposes. They want the benefits without the pain. They want us to believe them as they steal the truth. This is the aberrancy so many feel towards malingers. We vilify those who steal the truths, who want to benefit from that truth but without the prerequisite passage though the usual pains, sacrifices or discipline.[20] The same question arises again: Why can the person not survive with their own truths? Why do they need to steal the truth?

The mental health professional must replace any pejorative and vilipend "malingering labels" with explanations of the vilipend behaviors. That is often as important as offering a specific diagnosis. Many times the mental health professional is attacked by prosecutors in court for the assumption that in the "understanding" of a behavior is also a "suggested forgiving" of a behavior. What the prosecutors fail to see is that they are asking the mental health professional to be a judge and jury. That is not the role of the mental health professional. The court's job is to match the psychological truth of an individual's case with a suitable punishment. The hope is that the sentence will intimidate the person to change their ways or remove an uncontrollable person from society.

Someone suffering from a borderline or sociopathic personality disorder may appear to malinger symptoms in order to manipulate the situation. Indeed, those who interact with either of these disorders or malingerers will often feel negative emotions and frustrations because they are being asked to quickly solve problems that cannot be quickly fixed. They will often have the feeling that they are being used, and experience a sense of imposition. Most borderline personality disorder sufferers are actually very lonely and frightened people who are desperate for stable connections and relationships. They may not know how to maintain a good relationship or solve problems. Characteristically, they will blame others for their problems. That is a form of malingering, at least in style. It is not true malingering, however, because the borderline personality disorder is a full-time psychological vocation, whereas malingering is event specific. Nonetheless, a person suffering from borderline personality disorder might malinger in response to a specific event, which brings about an extraordinarily challenging and often fragile clinical picture to properly identify, classify and manage.

CHAPTER TWO

Shame and Malingering

Early and provident fear is the mother of safety.
~Edmund Burke~

The word *shame* has roots in the notion of hiding, covering, disgrace, and scandal. Two meanings of shame exist. It can be associated with shyness and bashfulness, or it can be associated with disgrace or scandal. Though often not immediately considered, bashfulness can be a reason for malingering.

Shame is a fear or displeasure that one's good image or self-respect has been compromised. Ashamed people regret or are afraid that others may have a negative opinion of them. Ashamed people often lack the ego structure to maintain a good self-image. They frequently feel psychologically disabled when faced with a "shameful situation." Shame is associated with "losing face," and, as such, they may experience inner anguish. Shame is also frequently associated with the process of keeping these feelings secret. The experiencing or fearing of shame can alter human behavior, and it can symptomatically range from mild hesitancy to unrelenting and disabling terror.

The concept of *losing face* is often tied to shame.[21] *Face*, as an idiom, is interwoven and coupled with a person's cultural thoughts about honor or humiliation. *Saving face*, especially in the Asian cultures, means that one is not being disrespectful to others in public. It often also connotes taking precautionary steps *not to lose face* in the eyes of others. One aspect of the *face* concept is that people often hide their faces when they are embarrassed or feel they are being looked at. Looking at a face can be emotionally powerful. It is how "we look into the person." The face is the garden and tattletale of nuances; indeed, no one nuance is as revealing as many nuances. Being embarrassed is losing the comfort in looking face-to-face with another person. This is why the nature of the facial contact between the suspected malingerer and other people is part of the diagnostic database.

Inherent in the concept of shame, and in the involvement of the idiomatic cliché of *saving face*, is the sociology within cultures of what causes shame and how to react to humiliation. Rosenberg discusses the notion of low and high context societies. The process of a psychological evaluation is essentially a form of negotiation as the evaluator seeks information from the subject. If the subject feels the potential loss of face as a very central issue, fear of shame can override the importance of revealing scientifically critical information. So the evaluator has to negotiate and set a comfortable table across which the negotiations can occur. Rosenberg writes that in Western countries the low-context society label applies. This means that verbal communication "is most often direct, and that there is very little concern or need for nonverbal cues in order for people to understand each other." She quotes another writer, Raymond Cohen, who believes that the "core of a low context society is the belief in the freedom of the individual, hence the term *individualistic* societies."

A *low-context* society's position is that individual rights supersede the commitments or affiliations to family, ethnic groups, or other community organizations. In other words, the individual is more important than the group. By extension, the low-context person would be less inclined to feel shame from a behavior because the values of the individual supersede the requirements of the society. Guilt is a personal event that acts as a "moral compass." If inappropriate behavior occurs as an adult, then no group shame results. Correcting a wrong may require only a private genuine apology or unseen self-introspection and change.

By contrast, *high-context* cultures, such as the traditional Oriental and Arabic cultures, emphasize group harmony. Being criticized by a group can produce deep humiliation and shame. In our Western society, falsifying data for economic, personal or political goals does not always result in group criticism. In fact, there are subtleties which reinforce falsification as a normal and expected way to achieve goals. The idea of a high-context society is captured in the *concepts* of our judicial system, but the bulk of social interactions never rise to the level where they interact with the judicial system. Consequently, shame in our society is more likely to be felt by being caught as opposed to feeling shame for committing the inappropriate behavior. Being caught in a lie is supposed to produce enough shame that the mere anticipation of that feeling would block behaviors that produce it. Certainly narcissistic and sociopathic personalities, by definition, would be less likely to feel shame and have less hesitancy to malinger.

For most people, shame is a normal reaction to guilt. The guilt can be for a crime or for an accidental failure of responsibility. If this was not so, then their community would be full of chaos. Many people are mixtures of low-context and high-context personalities.

Common sense would suggest that the fear of shame would prevent malingering. But the "public common sense" in our society is closer than not to the old saying, "do as I say—don't do as I do. But, if you do as I do, don't get caught."

Shame is often associated with how a person wishes to be viewed. "I am ashamed if I am not adequate or unique in the way I want to be unique." For example, someone who is indifferent to success as a musician would feel little shame if they could not play a piano. However, a seasoned accountant would feel shame for a serious and sloppy journal mistake.

Part of the understanding of an ego structure is knowing how a person deals with and learns from "shameful experiences" in their life. The role of shame in a person's life is therefore a critical diagnostic anchor; it reveals a great deal about superego and ego characteristics, and so it positions our approach to understanding their malingering.

If someone's ego structure is very frail or has experienced extensive and prolonged abuse, then the enormity of their shame serves as a portal into their superego. The only way to emotionally contend with this narcissistic superego is to diminish or remove oneself from the guilt; re-aligning oneself away from the responsibility for the guilt-producing event may be necessary.

An immature or skill-lacking ego might justify malingering to escape wicked superego attacks. If the person did someone wrong, or even if he was accused of doing something wrong, he may not be able to tolerate the shame of his situation. As such, malingering is primarily focused at removing himself from his own superego's punishment.

This malingering process is often focused on external matters, such as litigation. However, should the person be eventually exonerated by an external authority, such as the courts, then this same exoneration will cool down the superego attacks. The psychological motivations to malinger would be only partially understood if the fear and specter of superego punishments were not included in the explanation for the malingering.

Part of the malingering process is to remove oneself from a censoriously judgmental group. Malingering in a jail may win praise (the opposite of shame) from the other inmates. But if we usher both the malingerer and someone the malingerer respects into the same room, and expose the malingering, the malingerer may feel considerable shame. Malingering must be so tested by exposing the person to potential shame—doing so gives some real insight into the person's actual ego and supergo structure. For some people, their real worlds may be so dysfunctional that allowing a feeling of shame could be psychologically counterproductive insofar as their survival is concerned.

If there is no fear of superego punishment, then malingering behavior is more likely to derive from a strong narcissistic ego and a relatively impotent superego. This second set-up offers a motivation for malingering that is quite a different entity. Punishment is more of an inconvenience and annoyance to these people; it is not as psychologically deleterious as when a very strong superego is active. A weak or essentially inactive superego is much more suggestive of the antisocial personality disorder or malignant ego-based narcissism. The etiology of these weak or negligibly functioning superegos—which can manifest themselves with the absence of shame—may result from combinations of organic brain differences and life experiences which are just now being explored.

Metashame is when a person is too ashamed to admit that they are ashamed. Considered a sign of insecurity and as an inability to face others for fear of a harmful judgment, it is most often found in immature people. The person may fear such potential ridicule that they underreport their real feelings. It can also lead to malingering.

Shame is also provoked by the fear of being misunderstood— perhaps they fear that an embarrassing deficit will be highlighted. The falsifier will create information to try to be understood the way he wants to be understood. It is as much a "cover-up" of bad data as it is a "fill-in" with good data. This ties in with the potential of malingering or lesser confabulation.

Blushing is considered an automatic response to shame and embarrassment. I do not know if those who malinger blush more or less easily than others. It would be interesting to study if the presence of blushing—as measured by infrared face scans—indicates a propensity to malinger.

The biological origin of shame remains fascinating but inconclusive. No doubt our frontal lobe development is associated with ethics, but other cerebral functions, such as functional errors within the basal ganglia or other reward centers, may represent behavioral modules which account for the presence and differences between individuals and how they think and respond to the world. Frontal lobe pathologies are often associated with many behaviors that, but for an organic etiology, would otherwise be considered shameful. The mere (and hopefully healthy) maturation of cerebral circuitry, combined with psychological experiences, training, and the exposure (or lack of exposure) to chemically-toxic influences, all accumulate into the heart of an individual's overall style, psychological maturity and choices in life.

The ability to feel shame is an expected core aspect of our personalities. The common question — "do you feel no shame?"—carries amazement and disgust if the answer is "no, I don't feel shame." Like the narcissist, those who have no shame appear also to have no fears and no sensitivity to the suffering caused by their actions. Some would say that they have no *"yirat shamayin,"* (Hebrew for fear of God). Many malingerers feel no shame for the deception they present. They feel no shame for the harm caused by the actions which they are trying to explain away by their malingered pathologies. Those who have no shame, and those who have no shame in malingering, need to be assessed to determine if they feel a godlike power or if they report an association with God which exonerates them from human rules and strictures. Shame can be politically biased — someone may feel disgust at having to resort to causing the death of an enemy, but there may be no shame.

It is important to separate the malignant narcissist from the malingerer. The malignant narcissist genuinely believes that his position and authority in society supersedes the standard community's rules; he believes he has been given or earned elite powers and exemptions. In other words, he has a free pass.

The malingerer knows that he is feigning symptoms. The malignant narcissist may be reacting to a delusional system and so is not feigning symptoms. This aspect is similar to someone who is psychotic. Insofar as a pathology spectrum is concerned, the malingerer may be at an extreme and be more of a psychopathic. The narcissist is situated in the middle of this continuum, with the psychotic at the opposite pole from the psychopath. One differentiation may be visible following medication trials. The psychotic may improve while the psychopath would not.

The narcissist rarely responds to medication. The true narcissist does not willfully feign symptoms. The malingerer willfully designs the symptoms. The diagnostic challenge is, therefore, to separate these symptom clusters as clearly as possible.

It is also critical to understand the difference between a traditional narcissistic personality and the traditional malingerer. The narcissist lives a full-time lifestyle of putting themselves first and insisting that they be the center of attention. The narcissist may quite often blame others for problems and failures with projects; this is an all-encompassing personality strategy that does not vary with the situation. A narcissist can malinger in a specific situation, but on the whole, some fashion of malingering fits into the global style and politics of the narcissist as they go through life. The traditional malingerer uses malingering as a tactic to deal with a specific problem. Those who malinger do not have to be narcissistic, but they may use self-serving ploys when in trouble. The narcissist is self-serving even when there is no trouble.

Finally, it is also crucial to explore the differences between "narcissistic self-serving" or "malingering when in trouble" and "entitlement." Entitlement can have narcissistic underpinnings, but entitlement is not necessarily narcissism. The narcissist will say "I am owed something because I am special."

The entitled may want something but it is more an issue of being spoiled or immature. Entitlement is not always as pervasive or global in a person's life as is narcissism. The narcissist truly feels anointed or unique and may not feel shame. The entitled may not feel unique and may respond to rejection with hurt or fear and will feel shame. The narcissist responds to rejection with anger and rage. At the risk of being unscientific, I found it convenient and useful to call entitlement "narcissism-lite ." The entitled response to rejection—because rejection is a painful incident—may be converted into anger as a means of getting their way. It could also be a cover-up for the embarrassment of having an emotional weakness. The true narcissist will feel annoyance after rejection, but will never feel the emotional pain experienced by the entitled. Some people act as if they are narcissistic, but they are actually feeling entitlement only.

Those who malinger by design might be narcissists, feel entitled, or simply be so frightened that their usual repertoire of problem-solving skills has failed them. These skills are yet too weak or underdeveloped to resolve the problems before them. The narcissist does not shy away from the problems because his perspective on life exonerates him from any real responsibility. The entitled fears being responsible and guilty, is fearful of possible punishment, and just wants someone to take away the problem. The entitled fears that he may be forced to "own the problem," while the narcissist rejected the concept of "owning the problem" at the outset.

Therefore, the narcissist's use of malingering, if it occurs, evolves from a personality style to change the world to fit their needs. The narcissist may also shy away from malingering because to malinger might admit that they had some illness or flaw—narcissists blame others for problems. The narcissist would most likely use hierarchical malingering, not traditional malingering.

A good number of people who act narcissistic-like are, in fact, not true narcissists. They are bullies or they only act with a narcissistic style when around people they can intimidate. A true narcissist is almost impossible to intimidate. The narcissistic-like people have many narcissistic traits, but they lack the core of unshakeable self-love seen in the authentic narcissist.

Narcissists rarely feel shame. The entitled often feel shame. Most common malingerers, if they are caught, feel shame.

CHAPTER THREE

Malingering Styles

The physician is the servant of the art.
~Hippocrates~

Davidson[22] suggests that we have a single emotional dimension that builds on adaptive, albeit, primitive responses, which range from positive approaches to negative withdrawals. Similar dimension exists for malingering.

Malingering can fall into two styles: offensive and defensive. This assumes that the person is not delirious, metabolically compromised or psychotic.

Defensive malingering is done to protect oneself from harm in the manner of a child who does not know how to manage a problem. The child lies to remove himself from the problem. The action is more out of fear than a formatted or ingenious design. Any detailed plotting to pull together an exculpatory story falls apart easily under scrutiny. This malingering style is the product of immaturity, emotional or mental retardation, and fear. There is an important undercurrent sense of remorse, and the person can be taught that malingering is not good and cannot be accepted. This learning is best done by cognitive and insight-oriented therapy (pitched to the cognitive limitations of the person) and through persuasively significant positive and corrective emotional experiences. This malingering style comes from:

(1) poor problem-solving abilities for the current situation;

(2) lesser experience in the matters at hand;

(3) intellectual limitations and

(4) a great deal of fright or other incessantly disquieting emotions.

The defensive malingerer will likely want to be more than protected—he also might want to become a member of the doctor's or staff's emotional world. There is relatively little malignant ego functioning in the defensive malingerer. The ego function is more unskilled and immature than malevolent. Ultimately, he wants people to know him better. His actions may defy his real psychological make-up.

This defensive style is more also likely to be the consequence of Axis I and Axis IV stressors. Challenging a defensive malingerer will likely evoke fear and eventually shame.

Offensive malingering is a determined political process. It is a plot to deceive using carefully orchestrated symptoms that can—so it is hoped—resist and refute scrutiny. It is a willful desire to deceive and comes out of a faculty of excellent problem-solving abilities, good intellect, experience in the matters at hand, and fewer emotions. Remorse would be unlikely in the character make-up of the offensive malingerer. There is also less likelihood that this malinger will or can learn to change his ways. Excepting people with borderline personality clusters, this style is more a cluster B personality condition. Axis IV situations would much more likely trigger an Axis II response than an Axis I response. There are fewer "shame experiences" in the offensive malingerer's history. Challenging them will evoke anger, not fear. There is a considerable superego void and dysfunction. This malingerer does not want to be emotionally known outside of the boundaries in which he presents himself. Likewise, he does not want to move into the doctor's world. He does not want protection; he wants escape.

Challenging a defensive malingerer may also evoke anger, but the challenge is perceived as a threat. By contrast, the anger in a challenged offensive malingerer is perceived as an insult. Narcissism exists in the offensive malingerer—he feels that "I am smarter and know how to get away with this—even if I may need to have to redo my approach to outsmart them…"

The defensive malingerer says "I hope I can get away with this—how do I do that?." There is little or no narcissism in the defensive malingerer.

Clearly both offensive and defensive malingering produce grossly similar behaviors. They may give identical answers on a standardized test. But the primary motivational stems originate in very different personality structures. They are in fact two very different conditions but the current diagnostic schemes force them to be given the same label.

Serin[23] proposes a similar dichotomy in reference to types of violence: there is both a predatory and an affective violence. In concert with the strict liability notion, all violence is harmful and it simply cannot be tolerated. Predatory violence is characterized by a planned and emotionless violence. Affective violence is more reactive and defensive—it is characterized by some emotional reaction to the triggering events preceding the violence. Offensive malingering would more closely parallel predatory violence and defensive malingering would be more in line with affective violence.

Offensive malingering scripts tend to be more sophisticated than defensive scripts. Offensive script writers are more likely to have read some source document, like a psychiatry text, whereas the defensive malingerer may only have copied the symptoms or behaviors from others. This leads to greater inconsistencies in the defensive malingerer.

Real psychiatric patients in remission may merely replay their own former experiences from when their illnesses were active. But real psychiatric patients may also regress when under pressure or in fear. This is often when survival and problem-solving skills can be seen to be inadequate. They may malinger in some fashion in order to get help or feel safe. An example may be shyness. This is, of course, a social anxiety or phobia. Fears may be so prevalent or looming so massively in a person's mind that they malinger so as not to place themselves in the phobia-inducing environment.

Real psychiatric patients also have symptomatic fluctuations and can decompensate. Their conditions flux in and out of clinical and sub-clinical symptom manifestations. Anxiety and phobia sufferers are aware of situations which cause symptoms to appear. Women with pre-menstrual symptoms might also experience this, and they learn how to devote more ego activity to offsetting the potential impact of mood shifts when they are premenstrual. Borderline personalities may be more and less active, with behaviors that appear to shift. And certainly uncontrolled bipolar disorder shifts can change behaviors. How successful people are with controlling the effects of these shifts depends on their ego strengths, the intensity of the symptoms, the nature of psychological histories, and any limitation to other sets of problem solving skills.

In the past decades the psychiatric use of anticonvulsants as mood stabilizers has become very common. The anticonvulsants are being used in non-traditional seizure disorders, but there is on-going deliberation that these medications address low-level but real neuronal abnormal—and perhaps seizure—activity.

If someone was placed on a mood stabilizer and unwelcome psychiatric symptoms abated, the person is still left with a native intelligence, their psychological experiences, and their particular armamentarium of social skills.

I examined a young man who had been arrested for murdering his wife. He had a history of borderline personality disorder with frequent and short episodes of severe psychoses, frequent suicide attempts, and substance abuse. Several IQ tests gave him IQ scores in the mid-60s. He had never been treated aggressively with antipsychotics and mood stabilizers. I differed with many other mental health professionals who thought he was malingering. They felt his behaviors were not consistent over time. Fortunately a new prison psychiatrist began a course of aggressive psychopharmacology. The young man's mental status dramatically improved. He stopped cutting himself, he had more of an engaging presence, he became responsibly involved in unit activities, he was a little better able to assist his attorney, and he smiled more. The gross psychosis resolved, but his inventory of dysfunctional experiences and mental retardation remained. He had not been malingering. He had been psychotic. However, when the psychosis remitted, he better realized the full potential of the charges against him. But he was also so proud of how much better he was. Clearly someone who is happy to be better would not be a malingerer. He would have wanted to stay sick. The state hired several doctors who all felt he was malingering and competent, even before the medications had been started. It was amazing, however, that one of the doctors who saw him after the medications had been used felt that while he was competent, the medications were actually a placebo because in that non-medical doctor's opinion, he had always been competent. The doctor's opinion about the placebo was quickly challenged and rebuked because the quantity of medication the prisoner was taking was much too high to have placebo effects.

During my first meetings with the defendant, he said he killed no one and that people lied to him about the death. Then, after eight months of antipsychotic treatment there was comparatively very little focus on his illness. In fact, because the hallucinations were gone, and because he had a much better appreciation of the charges against him, it would have legally behooved him to maintain reports of illness, of appearing only partially responsive to treatment, and to say he was not much better. If he could have done it convincingly, then the murder charges might have been dropped because competency could not be obtained.

This same prisoner rolled a fecal ball on the table during an interview by a state-appointed examiner. The examiner arrived without an appointment. The examiner considered the prisoner to be malingering psychosis and depression. The questions that need to be addressed is how would the prisoner know to prepare the fecal ball in advance, especially if the fecal ball was never reported by nursing staff or mentioned in any other of many psychiatric evaluations? This is not offensive malingering because it is blatantly inconsistent across time.

His post-start-of-treatment behaviors were quite different, and it would have been too difficult for him to maintain an "act" all the time. This is a good example of how malingering is best diagnosed after a treatment trial.

There is a constitutional requirement that defendants must be competent to stand trial. This includes a capacity to assist their attorney and to sufficiently understand the nature of the proceedings so as to be able to actively participate in the legal process. This includes the ability to make unimpaired decisions about their rights, which includes an understanding of the ramifications of decisions they make or the decisions imposed on them by the courts. This has been called "decisional competence." The conventional standard has looked at mental illness as a cause of incompetence or disability, but realistically, a "maturity of judgment" is also required. Maturity of judgment is different than impairment of judgment. Age does not always predict maturity of judgment. The problem is not so much that a young teenager might be immature. The problem is when a thirty-five year-old is yet emotionally immature.

If someone chooses to malinger, the common assumption exists that they also understand, and have plotted, to use malingering as a device to manipulate the outcome of the situation. But what if someone malingers because they are emotionally more childlike than adult-like? Then the motivations for malingering might be very different. The childlike, emotionally immature malingerer may be engaging in more defensive malingering, whereas the more adult-like, emotionally mature malingerer is offensively malingering. The style of malingering is more significant than the presence of malingering.

Malingering, therefore, may be an indicator of non-permanent incompetence in emotionally immature people. The key therapeutic process in these situations is more a matter of "achieving," rather than "restoring" competence. Providing a defendant with access to good mental health care, including the availability and incorporation of a good social skill package and a decent support system, should help the malingerer "achieve" maturity such that malingering is no longer needed in his life.

Sometimes malingering has a predatory quality in that the malingerer wishes to spoil or even damage the examiner if he feels the examiner will not side with him. The offensive malingerer therefore intends to destroy the examiner's credibility by giving the examiner limited or faulty data and propaganda. By contrast, the defensive malingerer is asking for help in solving a problem. The defensive malingerer wants to be believed; he expends no energy in an effort to reduce the examiner's credibility. He wants the examiner to be his advocate.

The offensive malingerer, by comparison, will devote more energy plotting his malingering in an effort to intimidate or otherwise control the examiner; he wants the examiner to be his servant or minion. The defensive malingerer does not put as much conscious energy into designing a strategy. His malingering is much less politically sophisticated. The offensive malingerer is just the opposite. Psychotherapy may be able to help reduce future malingering in those who do it defensively. Psychotherapy is relatively ineffective with offensive malingerers. The defensive malingerer is likely to have a relatively strong superego with inadequate ego strngths. The offensive malingerer is more likely to have an ego much stronger than the superego.

CHAPTER FOUR

A Background and Historical Review

The trouble with people is not that they don't know
but that they know so much that ain't so.
~Josh Billings~

Factitious disorders[24], psychosomatic disorders, antisocial and borderline personality behaviors, and malingering are often confused or improperly blended.

The terms factitious (e.g., contrived, not natural, invented) and fictitious (e.g., conjured, fabricated, invented) have similar meanings, but the preferred and official term is factitious.[25] A factitious disorder is characterized by deceiving, lying, or undergoing diagnostic or surgical procedures for no apparent reason. Munchausen's syndrome is a factitious disorder. Factitious disorder patients often present with fantastic tales. There are marked inconsistencies in their stories; they have volumes of minute details of their medical illness but their lack of knowledge is unexpected and inconsistent with their experiences and details. It is distinguished from a malingering in that the patient wants to assume a long-term sick role.

A psychosomatic illness is one in which the emotional state of the patient significantly influences the scope and presentation of the reported illness. Commonly, this term is used to refer to patients and their disorders whose illnesses are believed to be, at least in part, secondary to psychological rather than physiological factors. Malingering breathes under this umbrella.

Common malingering has clearly definable goals that separate it from other fictitious disorders. The malingering goals usually fall into one of three categories:

(1) avoiding responsibility, punishment, or difficult or dangerous situations;

(2) to receive some sort of protection or compensation that might not otherwise be available to them unless they presented as being sick or

(3) to achieve some sort of retaliation against a person or entity which the patient claims caused the illness.

A regular diagnostic characteristic found in the malingerer is that the symptoms are vague, ill-defined and overly-dramatized. Malingerers often are preoccupied with compensation rather than cure. These external incentives are absent in factitious disorders. Malingering and factitious disorders do not result in symptom relief even with appropriate treatment for the proffered symptoms.

The nature of the doctor-patient relationship is critical to the diagnostic process and treatment of any disorder. If the doctor doubts the patient's integrity, the relationship is distorted and any future possible positive interactions between the patient and doctor are dangerously impaired. The doctor feels he is being asked to accept as natural something that seems patently unnatural. Treatment involves the further uncovering of relevant psychological or situational issues without being confrontational. A key diagnostic differential is the presence of a phase-of-life problem. The patient may lack the skills and mechanisms to properly deal with that specific presenting problem. Other problem-solving skills might or might not exist.

Malingering is usually not a unidimensional phenomenon. People malinger in response to their character make-ups, social issues and ego strengths. Because of this, data about historic and diagnostic overlaps are critical. A common overlap is the co-morbid presence of a personality disorder and malingering.

A widespread assumption is that malingering is not a unique abnormality, but rather a manifestation of a psychiatric illness. Psychiatric texts foster this confusion. For example, a common psychiatric textbook has a table entitled "Malingering features usually not found in genuine illness."[26] This is a misnomer and dangerously misleading because a genuine psychiatric illness is indeed causing these behaviors. This table does not rule out co-morbid psychiatric conditions, such as depression, psychoses, or borderline personalities.

Hutchinson[27] argues that the traditional motives assigned to malingerers do not explore the more central motivations. I agree. In order to "malinger," he says there must be deficiencies in the patient's object relations capacity and that the person must have very significant personality traits or disorders. Indeed, poor object relations may produce an inner anguish and a set of fears, such that, if coupled with poor problem-solving skills, could produce a decision to malinger.

An exploration of the person's sense of "I and Thou" could reveal a rich psychiatric library of the person's experiences and approaches to life.[28] The "I and Thou" and "I-It" concepts come from Martin Buber's exploration of a person's relationship to others and to a deity. One of the major themes of the book is that human life finds its meaningfulness in relationships. We cannot mention ourselves without an inference to either some "I-Thou" or "I-It" relationship. The level of analytic exploration required to do this usually exceeds the time and resources allotted to the evaluation for malingering. Or it may also be impossible to do because of other concurrent psychiatric disorders, lack of education, poorly-trained examiner skills and so on. Mirror neurons may explain some of this echoing, but if neurological research eventually discards the mirror neurons systems, nevertheless something triggers empathic resonations between people. We may not know how it happens, but we all know it does.

The question often asked is whether the malingerer is sick or wicked. The answer is not a binary or digital issue, but an analog one—degrees of simultaneous but varying threshold strengths of illness and wickedness are possible.

Empirical evidence does not generally support a link between malingering and antisocial personalities.[29,30] In the fifteenth century, patients who were considered insane were hospitalized at Bethlem Hospital in England. When they were discharged, they were given licenses to beg. Begging was officially illegal, but the licenses at least allowed these discharged patients to have some income. (This was the modern equivalent of being on disability.)

However, sane beggars began to feign insanity in order to get the license, so malingering flourished.

Several hundred years later saw the introduction of the term "moral insanity." This was applied to criminals and sociopaths. The implication was that a flaw in their morality resulted in their insane acts. There was no overt sense that these people were willfully sociopathic. The term was descriptive more than pejorative; there was perhaps a subtle inclination that these people could not control themselves, but the possibility of malingering was also tacitly understood.

Malingering is not limited to those in the criminal system. Indeed, malingering is far more common in the general population than most people may want to comfortably admit. Unfortunately, the term "malingering," has been used with the sloppy assumption that antisocial personality characteristics are necessary. Assuming responsibility for one's behaviors is a desired social ethic. There needs to be a means to measure the degree of malingering incidence and prevalence.

Proposing a rating scale of malingering intensity conjures up endless expectations of debates, but conceptually, we must clarify the dimensions between a white lie and a full lie. If we look at malingering simply as an effort to exonerate oneself from responsibility, then there is only one form of malingering. But if one malingers so as not to have to go out on a second blind date, then this malingering episode would rank closer to the white lie. This is different than malingering a psychiatric illness to avoid litigation. Every conscientious parent must walk a fragile line as they model to their children how to use white lies.

Sometimes the malingering motivation is quiet but very socially acceptable. That many civil litigations over-dramatize symptoms is an unspoken expectation. If this reflects some antisocial personality material, then the presence of accepted levels of dishonesty and sociopathy in our society is incredibly widespread.

During World War II, Sefton Delmer orchestrated a subtle British strategy towards the Germans known as Black Propaganda.[31] By 1942, the "black" propaganda section of the British Political Warfare Executive (PWE) printed booklets to help potentially malingering German soldiers and munitions workers to fake illness. The most famous version was *Krankheit rettet* – "Illness Saves by Doctor Do Good." Malingering instructions were in booklets, leaflets and even in cigarette paper packets. They were manuals on how to fake diseases. The intent was to convince Germans to avoid battle or hard or dangerous work without challenging a greater moral position. Delmer's manuals instructed people on how to fake throat infections to tuberculosis. A second intent was to make German commanders suspicious that soldiers claiming to be sick might indeed be healthy, so truly sick soldiers were sent to battle anyway. That would have had the felicitous dual effect of undermining the soldiers' commitment to their officers and spreading infectious diseases to uninfected soldiers.

The word psychopathology tries to differentiate between normal and abnormal psychic processes, with particular attention to socially accepted adaptive or maladaptive behaviors. A psychopath is considered to be a person who lacks both anxiety and guilt feelings about their behaviors. This term became more pejorative than helpful because "psychopaths" are found amongst some schizophrenics, the mentally retarded, and others in whom the indifference is not from a free will. The term has rather and sadly become associated with odd, erratic, impulsive, irrational or dangerous behaviors, despite the dissimilar purpose of these behaviors. It is similar to the legal separation between *acts rea* (an evil act) and *mens rea* (an evil intent).

Antisocial behaviors endanger the welfare of society. For many years prostitution was commonly considered an antisocial behavior. This was based on the violation of social norms, but it may not be a psychiatric disorder.

Diagnostically, adult antisocial behavior is listed in DSM-III-R as a condition not attributable to a mental disorder. Professional racketeers, thieves and swindlers are not considered to possess mental disorders, but they do endanger society and they are quite antisocial. However the DSM-IV gives adult antisocial behavior the status of a psychiatric disorder.

One difference between the antisocial, offensive malingerer and the defensive malingerer is that the former has lifelong goals, and not aims that are uniquely event-specific. These exceed the mere desire to survive—they want to design, shape, and ultimately control their entire environment. Large overlaps regularly exist between the offensive malingerer and the antisocial person. The defensive malingerer wants only to survive, is not concerned with ultimately controlling the environment, and will adapt to any situation to obtain that goal.

The DSM-IV-TR lists the prevalence rates for antisocial personality disorder in the general community at about 3% in males and 1% in females. Prevalence estimates within clinical settings have varied from 3% to 30%, and even higher rates are found in the prison settings.[32] Other authors provide similar numbers.

"It has been estimated, using DSM-IV-TR criteria, that 5.8% of men and 1.2% of women will merit the diagnosis of antisocial personality disorder during their lifetimes…"[33] Given a current census of about 300,000,000, the prevalence of antisocial personalities in the United States is between 1,200,000 and 2,100,000 people. No statistics could be found which suggest how many malingers exist among those 300 million, but it is probably much larger.

Goodwin and Hamilton[34] describe some interesting aspects of the antisocial personality (ASPD). "Overall, 3.3% of the population has ASPD (lifetime), 9.4% had conduct disorder without ASPD, and 23.9% had an anxiety disorder without ASPD…. Social phobia and post-traumatic stress disorders were associated with significantly increased odds of ASPD." Then they question: "…if…severe anxiety is associated with increased likelihood of antisocial behavior and ASPD."

This was an epidemiologic study, so this is a quantitative, not a qualitative study, but it is an intriguing finding.

A "choice" implies some element of free will, with the presence of a design and planning, frontal lobe maturation and lack of other impairing brain dysfunctions. It also suggests a conscious organization that can be objectively tested as knowingly in violation of a social code. Some—not all—behavior comes from free will.

Free will is supposed to endow the ability to choose between right and wrong. The pivotal word is "ability." Given no medical impairment, or no unwanted outer, coercive or corrosive force, then the will to choose is free. But practically speaking, no choice can separate from the full force of a person's lifelong experiences preceding the choice.

Geiger[35] provides an excellent study of Israeli Mizrahi women who have malingered. She suggests that explaining that their malingered insanity "has been interpreted as purposed actions initiated by agents to struggle against abusive and oppressive conditions…These women often are simply acting as free agents asserting their will to resist." One woman "freaked out and was placed in an institution for the mentally ill to escape her abusive brother who wanted to reduce her to mere sexual property."

The girl acted as she did because she had to assume a different role to survive. This would be defensive malingering, and in this situation, it is not an evil thing to do. It would also be interesting to know if that subset of Mizrahi women who drifted into crime and prostitution had some promoter genetic defect similar to the MAO-A polymorphism found in young boys.

Is there a theory explaining why one chooses evil rather than good? Religious thought can help. Interestingly, the process is very consonant with psychodynamic theories.

Deuteronomy 30:15-19 says:

See, I have set before you today life and good, and death and evil; in that I command you today to love the Lord your God, to walk in His ways and to keep His commandments and His statutes and His judgments, that you may live and multiply, and that the Lord your God may bless you in the land where you are entering to possess it. But if your heart turns away and you will not obey, but are drawn away and worship other gods and serve them, I declare to you today that you shall surely perish. You will not prolong your days in the land where you are crossing the Jordan to enter and possess it. I call heaven and earth to witness against you today, that I have set before you life and death, the blessing and evil. So choose life in order that you may live, you and your descendants.

The unambiguous instruction in this passage is that by avoiding evil, one avoids premature death and can achieve salvation. It also suggests that we have the free will to choose life. Deuteronomy has been called the book of obedience and the "follow the law" book.[36]

Evil causes death to something. Death will remove or avoid pain. Biblically, death refers to both an escape (symbolically) from the pains and stresses in life and from life itself. No problem is solved by choosing evil. Problems may appear to be eliminated or unaddressed when evil is chosen. The movement away from the obligatory addressing of a problem could be a form of death to those depending on the problem to be solved. Choosing evil reduces or removes the ability to achieve any lasting personal greatness, though it may produce short term freedoms or fame.

True merit and honest growth branch out from how we work out conflicts. We must use our free will to grow and not die, to not quit, to tackle reality and avoid escapes. To choose life is to embrace personal responsibility. To be indifferent to the "life" and to routinely choose "evil" are components of an antisocial personality. Typically, these people choose short-term gains that have no potential, long-term, to enhance life.

Yet, the same nagging question begs our attention: what process forces or directs a person to embrace attitudes that make them choose evil over good?

Scientists view free will somewhat differently.

The definition of free will, as it is traditionally understood, needs modification. The neurological structures which determine a behavioral choice must be understood in a manner that still allows for social responsibility. Clear evidence exists that brain peptide density in non-human mammals has been associated with monogamous or polygamous relationships—male prairie wolves with high density vasopressin binding sites are monogamous, while those with low density binding sites are polygamous.

In humans, the peptide oxytocin is associated with mother-child bonding. The oxytocin binds to the receptors that reinforce the bond. Obviously, these behaviors are influenced by the quantity and nature of the binding sites as well as the availability of the peptides—someone could have the "normal" number of receptors but not have the peptide. The differences can change behavior. The basis of the behavior is, therefore, genetic or evidence of some disease process.

People with tumors might present with unusual behaviors. This is conceptually identical to a penny resting across electrical contacts in a computer—the circuit board is shorting. And the information about the MAO polymorphisms might also suggest a reason for aberrant behaviors.

A rigid stance and definition of free will is that the decision is "uncaused." A truly "free will" choice has no influence in persuading the person to employ a history of prior experiences or knowledge in the decision-making process. Free will means the decision is completely independent of the person's life, biases, education, chemistry, etc. This is, of course, not the way our brains function.

We go from one mental state to the next. Any non-delirium decision is the sum of all antecedent conditions faced with new environmental challenges—the mental process then computes and exacts a decision which anticipates a future. Such computations may employ more of the prefrontal cortex than other areas of the brain, but the prefrontal cortex is heavily influenced by countless other brain areas offering their own expectations, experiences and editorials. This process is also highly influenced by the computing program, which reflects and is the result of education and social experiences. No one sees a computer as having free will. It operates within the boundary of the nature of its memory and processor, the nature and bias of the computing code, its operating temperature and degree of insulation from dangerous extraneous electromagnetic manipulators, and the nature and bias of the database. Free will assumes an unlimited resource base; having a restricted base means the will to choose is not truly free.

Free will is perhaps better conceptualized as styles of self-control. I believe there is no truly free will, but only an "optional will" or a "will of consideration" which reflects the summation of past experiences. The optional will is the organization and resources with which the person creates a tactic in response to a particular problem.

I once heard that we "all have a unique set of "make-sense of the world" neurotools. These tools are like muscles, growing in the style of how they are prepped and used."

The stiff-necked neuroscientist or religious believer may declare that all behaviors are outgrowths of all prior experiences or moral inclinations. It does not matter because the origin is not as important as is the maintenance of some social order. It does matter, however, if we want to prevent destructive behaviors. People act to survive, and choosing the methods to survive is the product of the will.

An unsullied and free will does not exist outside of some disease states in which no history can influence a choice. Indeed, such a situation would be better labeled as a random will, not free will. If it was free, then there would be an ability to enhance survival. Random will endangers survival.

Our egos enjoy the feeling that we are free-willed, but that is not accurate. The free will hypothesis proposes that we are free, and it releases us from external determinism. Our inborn DNA offers us a copy of software that is an ever-evolving and improved survival recipe. And our genetic footings present with different phenotypes, which become variations in the software and hardware that help us learn to better survive as a species. Free will would not need these variations to survive. Free will does not need evolution, growth, trial and error, or teaching; it might not make mistakes. Free will is not instinctive; people have to be taught how to use their free will. Free will therefore fluctuates in character with how the person was educated, etc. Free will is therefore an illusion.

Try to consider the task of designing a flawless machine to make truly "free willed" decisions. No machine could be programmed with every possible alternative. The software itself would introduce peculiarities that skew any result. It would have to be an electromechanically perfect machine with perfect software, working in a perfect environment. A machine designed to figure out how to survive would have to have some sense of how it wants to survive, and making that choice has to be based on some understanding of the relative merits and handicaps of making one choice over another. Where would it get that information from?

A universally perfect machine needs untainted data. But the untainted quality would exist for just the first decision the machine has to make. Follow-up decisions need the success or failures of the first decision as a lesson of what works and what does not.

The central query is how to explain why non-diseased people choose behaviors that are clearly contrary to the normal or expected social codes. The answer is unexpectedly simple—their behavioral choices reflect what they feel they need or deserve to survive. Malingering is first and foremost an individual's survival technique. An offensive malingering individual is unsympathetic to the larger ramifications of his lie in the context of the larger social system in which he lives. The defensive malinger wants to join that larger social system.

As such, offensive malingering can be defiantly irritating, tormenting, and a relentless burden to a social system.

There is a difference between "antisocial behaviors and choices" and what I call *unsocial* choices or behaviors. The *antisocial behaviors* are contrary to social code expectations, but these can also be motivated by retaliations—this implies a conscious rejection or disregard of the community code of behavior. The *unsocial choices and behavior* would be motivated by an indifference to social codes. The antisocial acting person may, in fact, have an emotional affiliation with the social code and may actually want to be applauded by that code, but for various reasons, that code frustrates him, so he acts out and usually gets into trouble. The *unsocially* acting person has no emotional affiliation or empathy for that code; this is akin to malignant narcissism and it is a very dangerous personality in most communities. Antisocial personalities are usually labeled as lacking remorse and being cold-hearted. However, the majority of antisocial personalities I have known do display some feeling and emotional pain. And when the conditions are in alignment, they can show signs of kindness and concern. The unsocial person is devoid of any caring emotions other than emotions which serve his own pleasures.

The eighteen-year-old uneducated male cannot find a job but wants to be successful in the eyes of his girlfriend. He knows drug dealing is wrong, but he knows there will be great applause from many peer sources if he has money. He feels frustrated in his society but feels justified in violating some aspects of society's code—namely marketing illegal drugs—to achieve what he believes is a higher position of success in his society. This is antisocial behavior.

A mob leader felt no hesitation at physically harming people who did not pay him his protection fees. But he would cry and feel deep empathy for family members who were sick, and he would give charity to the church, send poor kids to camp, sponsor school trips, etc. He had aspects of unsocial and antisocial behaviors.

I interviewed a prisoner who was charged with raping a paraplegic woman. I asked him if he had any feelings for the victim, of what she might have felt. His response demonstrated an absence of sensitivity and compassion. He told me, "isn't that what women are for?" This is unsocial behavior.

The unsocial person has no empathy for the social or religious customs of an ethnic group and feels no hesitation or shame by invading their homeland. The unsocial actor imposes his social code on his victims and does not share any commonality with his victim's social code. If there are some similar codes with the victim, the unsocial actor might exploit aspects of this overlap in order to gain some mastery over the victim. This is often called competition. The unsocial actor, however, is not competing. The unsocial actor is not interested in sharing the world with his victims, other than perhaps by enslaving them. Because both the antisocial and the unsocial characters can be so disruptive and contrary to a society's peaceful existence, they are both clustered under the notion of behavior against the society and its code.

The historically common preface to this behavior would use the prefix "anti-." Hence, the notion of antisocial behavior. However, the term "antisocial" is now so widely used that it has become overly generalized. As such it does not reflect some of the motivational differences inherent in the behaviors labeled as antisocial. An antisocial behavior may, in fact, be motivated by a desire to be like the victim, or to assume his position in society. The unsocial behavior has no interest in being like the victim. The unsocial may absolutely destroy to get his goal, but the antisocial will consider what spoils or systems might be important to save in order that the conquered system could still be productive.

A corporate vice-president felt he had been unfairly bypassed for promotion. He therefore began circulating clandestine and nefarious rumors to discredit his boss's integrity. He did not want to change the basic corporate organization, but simply to become the leader of the corporation. He wants to be at the top of the shared social code. Lying and malingering occurred. This is antisocial behavior.

By contrast, the religious zealot wants to take over an adjacent country. He wants not only to rule the country, but also to impose a completely new social code consistent with his own values. He is indifferent to, and felt no obligation to maintain the community traditions of the land he wants to conquer. If captured and jailed, there is no need to lie or malinger, other than to stay alive long enough to return to power or to escape back to return to one's war room. This is unsocial behavior.

An interesting analogy comes from the types of weapons an army can use. Conventional bombs hit narrow targets. A munitions factory may be targeted, but adjacent bridges are preserved because the army needs them. Nuclear bombs, however, wipe out and destroy everything. It attacks life itself, and it destroys both for the immediate war and for years thereafter. The nuclear bomb is an *unsocial weapon*. Tradition weapons are *antisocial*.

The unsocialized actor will not benefit from rehabilitation. They see no need to change. The antisocial actor could theoretically benefit from rehabilitation. Although the terms "psychopath" and "antisocial personality" are often commonly confused because of the many connotative overlaps, the psychopath is more fundamentalistic and narcissistic in his make-up. In the context of this discussion, the psychopath may fall under the umbrella of unsocial behavior. The psychopath's gross behaviors may appear antisocial, but the motivation is unsocial. Meloy reports that psychopaths do not respond to treatment and may even worsen in spite of treatment.[37]

Other writers have reached the same conclusion:

The fundamentalists, by "knowing" the answers before they start, and then forcing nature into the straitjacket of their discredited preconceptions, lie outside the domain of science—or of any honest intellectual inquiry. ~*Stephen Jay Gould,* Bully for Brontosaurus

Such a differentiation would suggest that antisocial behaviors, as defined above, would rank more as a psychopathology. Unsocial behavior, therefore, falls more into the realm of a moral choice. The question is, however, why would someone make a unperturbed moral choice knowing that it would be so disruptive to other people? Where is the sense of respect and empathy for the potential victims? And what role does the victim play in the unsocial actor's life? Such inquiries are vigorously debated and rarely adequately answered. There is, however, attractive and compelling logic to the idea that the unsocial person is frequently the result of severe childhood trauma. Neurological flaws which limit empathy might also be at play.

He who is unable to live in society, or who has no need because he is sufficient for himself, must be either a beast or a god. ~Aristotle~

Meloy[38] believes that "…wickedness, or evil, is outside the paradigm of science, and I think, should remain so. It is, instead, the default of morality, or moral choice, it occupies the paradoxical position of being known to the science of psychology, yet not of it." Nonetheless, he does reference data that habitual criminality has a genetic genesis.

Evidence does suggest a biological link between antisocial behavior and a short variant of the MAO-A (monoamine oxidase A) gene.[39,40] The combination of this genetic variant with harsh discipline, physical abuse and other forms of maltreatment puts young men at a greater risk of antisocial behavior. MAO-A is an enzyme that metabolizes neurotransmitters that are involved in stress and moods. The shorted gene variant is thought to make these youngsters more vulnerable to the effects of maltreatment. It may trigger anxiety, impulsivity, aggression or other reactions to being besieged. Of course, given the variant, the question remains, "Will these youngsters have heightened negative and abnormal responses to more or less normal levels of criticism and stresses in life?"

So where does malingering belong? Is it the product of psychopathology or is it the product of religious and philosophical aberrations? Should its management and cure (if possible) belong to clergyman, legislators, parents, psychotherapists or neuroscientists?

Or is malingering an evil thing to do? Does it stem from the magical fancy of evil? There is a thrilling aspect of evil—it draws us to look at it. Somehow we all know a little bit about it; it gives simple answers. And, come what may, there is a delightful taste to some levels of evil. Evil is the apple in the Garden of Eden.

Evil can probably be most accurately described as a willingness to act in opposition to the best interests, desires and needs of other people. When those evil acts occur, it causes suffering. Evil, in the larger scope of human experiences, is something which ought not to exist. Evil is felt when an undesirable force is directing behaviors away from those which are wanted. The key factor is when an outside influence—unwanted, destructive, and alien to the victim's chosen style of life—crashes into and oppresses that person's life. A sense of crime follows when someone asks others to believe a false (i.e., malingered) set of symptoms or data. People who make us feel that way are customarily labeled as evil or wicked.

Evil implies the imposition of suffering. Evils include bodily injury, sickness, danger, poverty and oppression, and mental suffering. Understandably, seeking an explanation for the origin of evil has produced a wide number of opinions. Certain themes exist, however. Those who perform evil do so with the intent of depriving others of something necessary for their lives. A good indicator of evil is the degree of pain experienced by the victim. Evil is regarded as perverse because it rejects associations and choices based on mutual respect and wellbeing.

Like lying and deception, evil has a relative quality to it, but this is a matter of situational interpretation and often arises from a misuse of the word "evil." A child may consider a parent evil if the parent insists on placing the child under some behavioral restraint. This is, of course, not evil since the intent of the action is to benefit the "victim." Evil is implicated when the evildoer is either indifferent to the pain he causes or rejoices in the pain he is responsible for. If a parent commits "evil," but has great empathy and displeasure in the pain felt by his action towards his child, then this would not be evil.

Those who malinger are not necessarily evil; some may indeed feel the pain of those who suffered from their actions. The malingerer merely wants to be exonerated. The psychopath or the malignant narcissist, on the other hand, is considerably less likely to feel any compassion or remorse for the suffering caused by his actions. Although those who malinger may share psychopathic, sociopathic and narcissistic traits, these groups do not automatically overlap. A psychopath may malinger, but the typical malingerer is not likely to become a psychopath.

Morris Adler[41] offers this observation:

The word "good" in the Biblical verse "…and God saw everything that He made and behold it was very good." (Genesis 1.31) includes the evil as well as the good impulse. But, it is asked, how can the evil impulse be termed "good?" The answer is "were it not for that impulse a man would not build a house, marry a wife, beget children or engage in trade."

"Thou shalt love the Lord thy God with all thy heart." (Deuteronomy 6.5) means with evil and good impulses (hence with *all my heart*). Even the evil impulse can be used in the service of God.

The evil impulse leads a man astray in this world and testifies against him in the next. The evil impulse within man seeks to restrain him from charitable acts by saying, "why practice charity and reduce your possessions? Rather than give to strangers, give to your children."

"There shall be no strange god in thee." (Psalm 81.9). Who is the strange god in man? It is the evil impulse.

Accepting this observation as a true characterization of human nature helps us recognize that the chance of evil-doing is a fundamental human propensity.

Understanding human choices is similar to watching moving clouds. Clouds move because of winds and weather systems thousands of miles away. We also know that weather systems are also influenced by such things as volcanic eruptions, sunspots, and human contributions to global warming. The hurricane passing over Florida today is the product of yesterday's weather in Africa. We may want to deal with local weather as a single storm, but to understand how to predict, and perhaps, how to prevent dangerous weather, we need to study global influences. The destruction and "evilness" of a horrible storm is the outgrowth of a worldwide series of faraway benign events.

This analogy can epitomize most human behavior—evil actions are the outgrowths of historical events. But how to explain evil in the absence of problematic psychosocial historical events? Is evil inborn? Perhaps so, especially if an untroubled psychosocial history is overruled by either traceable genetic tendencies, new disease or a *de novo* genetic abnormality. Acting evil represents how the brain—our computer, if you will, operates. It is an erroneous presumption that every computer's hard and software is harmless.

The next question is: why do people need to be evil? What underlying manifestation in a psychological makeup obscures the usual approach and respect for our painfully expensive and evolved social systems? One interesting thought is that it makes no sense for evil to exist since all of us are parts of the same cosmic process. We all share the same ultimate fate and need the same materials for survival and procreation—yet we war against each other.

Is evil simply nature's method of preventing a lackadaisical approach to life? Does the fear of evil spur a drive to develop and protect ourselves? If God is all-benevolent, then why is suffering permitted? If evil is the product of illness, such as sociopathic personality disorders, then why does a God permit the existence of illness? There is a chilling quality to the hypothesis that evil is good for us because it serves to induce behaviors to insure our own existence. Buddhism claims that the origin of suffering is the "thirst for being." Greek philosophers tell us that life was valueless and that pleasure was unattainable. They felt that evil is supreme but can be overcome or avoided by the virtuous and wise. Some describe evil as the absence of good, such as the hole in a good donut.

Suffering may be a product of our own self-consciousness, which seeks a level of happiness that may not be obtainable. Perhaps those who act evilly are less able to enjoy the usual emotional and social comforts. They feel the need to aggressively control their own environment, to feed only themselves, so to speak, and to focus single-mindedly on their own happiness. As a society, we feel a danger from evil orientations; we build social systems to avoid the selfishness of evil, since a safe society cannot exist on a foundation defined by selfishness and evil.

Evil might be considered revenge. A child, being the product of horrific abuse, may be so angry at the world that their evil behaviors are only symbolic expressions from their emotional core, seeking out some level of balance with life. Indeed, this very old observation is what brings us to the stem cell equivalent of psychiatric research. Research has shown that children with genetic inheritances, who live in certain types of environments, are more likely than not to become antisocial.[42] The research authors clearly noted that there had to be a combination of the low-MAO

A gene activity and environmental maltreatment in order for the development of the antisocial behavior to occur.

Even children from the same family do not necessarily get the same parenting. Parents have their own emotional fluctuating needs, and there may be external economic or other forces distracting parents from their children at different times in their different children's lives. And, of course, the genetic make-ups, though very close, are only approximate from child to child. There tend to be less psychotherapeutic interventions with the caregivers when a child is having a problem—the focus tends to focus therapeutically on the child. The possibility that parenting changes might actually alter how genes are expressed in vulnerable children was supported by a fifteen year-long study that found that repeated home visits by nurses resulted in children who had fewer rates of antisocial behaviors.[43] It appears that the nature or nurture questions are not separate and dichotomous processes, but are truly enmeshed.

By the same token, neurological abnormalities unrelated to understandable genetic influences can cause changes in behavior. For example, amygdala hyperactivity has been associated with misreading facial cues. This leads to hypervigilence.[44] That can drive a person to engage in socially undesirable actions.

Christian and Hebrew philosophies contend that man brought evil unto himself by not following God's laws. The pain from evil therefore contributes to the eventual perfection of mankind by giving people the reason to act in a certain manner. Evil is merely the absence of goodness. Therefore an evil can be eradicated by a goodness.

An interesting thought amongst many people is why God allowed evil to exist. After all, we are the ones who suffer and feel pain because of that decision. The answer is often overshadowed by the concept that we do not understand the larger cosmic plan. Perhaps our pain is beneficial to some other aspect of the plan. It brings us to the unsolved mystery of creation.

Religion has been vigorously challenged by those who feel pain. The challenge questions God's wisdom and mercy. If God made evil, or allows it to exist, why could God not change things to help us suffer less? One notion is that God cannot change His mind since to do so would show that He had a defect in his decision-making process. Many believe God gave us free will and that evil is our misuse of free will. Should God therefore be held accountable for miscalculating how we would use free will? This would be an acknowledgment by God that He is not all-knowing and all-powerful. The topic of evil, therefore, can only be gingerly addressed because to question why there is evil in our lives is to question the wisdom and sanctity of creation. Evil, therefore, exists not because of God's doings, but rather, our failures. The malingerer, therefore, is seen as someone who chooses to use deception from the inventory of available free will behaviors. His choice of behaviors is contrary to goodness and honesty, which is, by definition, evil. Therefore, the malingerer is considered by many to be a failed and non-virtuous person.

The psychiatric task is to identify why a malingered behavior was selected.

The Bible reports that King David feigned mental illness, "And he changed his behavior before them, and feigned himself mad in their hands. He scratched on the doors of the gate and his spittle fell down upon his beard." [45] Scholars question the utility of David's feigned mental illness. They ask, "what purpose does a madman serve?" The Midrash answers by a saying, "you wish to contest the usefulness of insanity? By your life, he shall have need of it!" During David's flight from King Saul to the King of Gath, the truth of this teaching became apparent.

One often comes across the teaching in antiquity which states that a criminal is ill in his soul. "A person does not commit a transgression until a spirit of folly enters into him…thus a woman only commits adultery if she becomes mentally deranged. (The Sages were asked) if God derives no satisfaction from idolatry, why does He not destroy it? They answered: if people would only idolize useless things, then God would in fact destroy them. However, they also idolize the sin, the moon and the stars. Should He destroy the world because of fools?"

Kornfeld asserts that "in the Bible, crimes and psychic disturbances are fundamentally separated from each other… unruly or violent madmen were simply put into chains…until Pinel (in 1795)." [46]

Behavioral abnormalities seem to have existed from the dawn of history and across all human societies. On the whole, the ancients regarded mental abnormalities as having a supernatural origin. In a sense, then, modern mental health efforts have been concerned with the gradual freeing of our psychological concepts from that being controlled by a supernatural force to the recognition of our current biopsychosocial explanations. Indeed, Hippocrates, in the fifth century BC, preferred to call epilepsy a physical disease and not a sacred one. He also believed that mental disease was regulated by brain functions. Furthermore, he felt that mental abnormalities did not separate themselves from normal in a hard and fast manner, but through a series of gradations.

Later, physiologists in Alexandria felt that behavior was related to the nerve functions. Galen, in about 200 AD, examined a woman with severe anxiety that did not have an obvious physical cause. He studied her case and noticed that when a particular man's name was mentioned, her pulse rate went up. His diagnosis was that she was in love and could not admit it.

After the fall of the Greek and Roman civilizations, and the invasions throughout Europe of barbaric tribes, civilization fell into the "dark ages." Demonic interpretations of behavioral abnormalities were common. The supernatural was once again in control of abnormal behaviors. As the concept of personal devils evolved, it was easy for people to simplistically explain unusual behaviors as the product of the devilish invasions which demolished and took control of the soul. Treatment, therefore, became the "casting out of the devils and the acceptance of God."

When these abnormalities existed, they were labeled as "devil sickness."

In 1621, Burton [47] wrote the *Anatomy of Melancholy*. This was one of the first works that studied the different forms of insanity.

Syndeham, in 1692, wrote *Processus Integri*.[48] He offered a set of relatively objective descriptions of mental abnormalities. Syndeham's work is a seminal study of mental disorders because it considered and offered objective classifications of types of abnormalities. He did not merely attribute behavioral abnormalities solely to an invasion of misfortunes or the devil.

It was not until the 18th century that the French psychiatrist, Pinel, introduced a very humanitarian categorization of the mentally ill. He is credited with saying that patients are not wicked—but they are sick.

For many years, the primary research into abnormal behaviors was done by physicians, not psychologists. Psychologists tended to focus more on considerations of measuring intelligence. Moreau de Tours, a psychologist, is credited with the beginnings of a psychological approach to mental illness, writing that behavioral abnormalities can result from psychological processes. In the latter half of the nineteenth century, Charcot and other psychologists devoted much work to the theories of suggestion and hysteria. This led to early but intriguing formulations of the unconscious and dissociation. By the late nineteenth century, Freud began his remarkable work.

Concurrently, the school of thought associated with Pavlov explored a principal of behavior and learning associated with numerous ways in which we adjust our lives to our environments. The notion of conditioned responses can explain many behavioral abnormalities and problems. Combining the seminal works of the Freudian and Pavlovian schools gives us powerful concepts with which to explain a behavior's origin and symbolic meanings. At first reflection, these may seem to be separate processes. But experience has shown us that biochemical abnormalities can influence a psychological environment, which, in combination, can then cause abnormal behaviors. Likewise, repeated or traumatic psychological traumas influence and disrupt a normal biochemical environment.

Hart[49] perceptively observes that many of the symptoms of insanity are conditions known to many normal people but they differ in the insane due to their intensity and the lack of any cause. The symptoms are different than normal because they are not just exaggerated, but distorted and senseless. At the extreme, when we consider incomprehensible hallucinations and delusions, the immediate similarities to a normal person is harder to find. Hart says, "yet we shall find as we proceed but even the most bizarre symptoms are not so very different from processes to be discovered in our own minds, and that the lunatic appears more and more like ourselves the better we are able to penetrate into the torturous recesses of his spirit,..." He alludes that certain levels of insanity result from the associations and he offers the following definition: "A system of ideas is said to be dissociated when it is divorced from the personality and when its course and development are exempt from the control of the personality." Malingering is a symptom of exerted control in the personality.

By extension, therefore, the suspicion of malingering would have to be tested against the backdrop of how much control the alleged malingerer genuinely has over those aspects of his personality which control the questionable (and possibly malingered) behaviors. If the motivation is truly "divorced" from the core personality, then an insanity explanation may exist. If the motivation is an integral part of the core personality, then the next diagnostic test should determine if this is offensive or defensive malingering. The true malingerer does so out of a psychodynamic process and interaction with his world. Malingering would be considered a mental disease, not a brain disease.

Many years ago, the concept of dissociation would have been used to explain uncontrollable behaviors that happened with the person's full awareness of the actions. Today this might be seen within the spectrum of an obsessive-compulsive disorder. Hart discusses the lady who becomes intolerably distressed at her own "foolish behavior"—if she was trying to defend a behavior that resulted in some legal action, it would have to be explained by the notion of an irresistible impulse, at a minimum level, and insanity at a maximum level. The behavioral phenomena needs two explanatory parts: first, the etiology of the behavior, and second, a true measure of how much control the person had in being able to keep the psychological drives contained within the limits of socially acceptable behaviors. Likewise, there is a continuum of impulses, running from a melody that will not leave one's mind or an irresistible impulse to check the locks. The person is cognizant of the force driving them to do it, and, although it may be familiar to a person's core of psychology, its presence is painful.

To the affected person, our objective scientific arguments about the improbability or impossibility of their concerns is frequently received with an acknowledgment that they cognitively understand our arguments, but the arguments do not penetrate into their psychological logic enough that the symptoms are reversed or removed. Aggressive cognitive therapy works against this very challenge. By and large, the non-malingerer willfully engages and will get some level benefit from therapy. The malingerer will not even seriously engage in intensive and challenging self-explorations done for the purpose of therapy.

The psychoanalytic notion of repression may play a role in malingering . Repressing a painful experience may become a psychological survival technique. This could explain malingering in that the person chooses to deflect approaches and challenges that might resurrect emotional pain. Portraying feigned symptomatology to distract others from his real psychological mental state is defensive malingering. Once the psychological history is known, it becomes possible to reconstruct the processes responsible for the exhibited symptoms. For example, people who feel a deep deficiency or a self-perceived fault of which they are ashamed may work very hard to keep that hidden. Alcoholism frequently appears in these people, and alcoholism has been characterized as one of the great refuges away from life and its stresses. Occasionally, a person will feverishly protect their own ego by projecting responsibility for their actions, and their errors, onto other people or agencies.

This might present as a paranoia or delusional system. Some of the important elements in understanding these behaviors include a study of childhood psychopathology and how the person was prepared for adulthood.

The concept of hysteria is related to malingering. Hysterical reactions are now known as conversion disorders, hypochondriasis and other somatic form disorders in which the symptoms presented are incompatible with known physiologic disease patterns. On the surface, these might be factitious disorders. These are often associated with antisocial and histrionic personality disorders, perhaps obsessive-compulsive disorders, or even psychological immaturity and mental retardation. Diagnostically, differentiating a somatoform disorder from malingering requires a careful analysis of the person's psychological makeup before the event occurred— before the malingering.

Science must combine all these contemporary theories to try to create a proper origin of the abnormality.

Mental disease is not yet sufficiently separated from that which is called a "brain disease" and from that which is the "mental disease." The latter has been anchored to the fundamental personality characteristics of the person and may be the expression of the deepest fantasies and wishes. The brain disease camp, in its purest sense, is not influenced by the personality. The diagnostic challenge is obviously to make and accurately proportion the influences. The same diagnostic challenge requires that the influences be given etiologies as best as contemporary knowledge will allow.

So, are those who malinger:

(1) legitimately psychiatrically sick;

(2) psychologically immature;

(3) from a different culture or have a series of distinctive social experiences;

(4) morphologically have immature or dysfunctioning brains;

(5) morally impaired or indifferent, or

(6) healthy opportunistic profiteers gainfully engaging in an accepted and prevalent social code?

It could be one, or a mixture, of any of these.

Hugo Münsterberg

Nearly one hundred years ago, Hugo Münsterberg, a professor of psychology at Harvard University, published a book entitled "On The Witness Stand—Essays on Psychology and Crime."[50] It is a fascinating essay and so rich in historical data. It is also a great tour of how other people dealt with the same problems that we encounter today. One of his chapters looks at how to measure the Traces of Emotions. It would be remiss for this essay not to acknowledge his work. Here are selected excerpts from his 1908 treatise:

To make psychology serviceable cannot mean simply to pick up some bits of theoretical psychology and to throw them down before the public. This has sometimes been done by amateurish hands and with disastrous results. Undigested psychological knowledge has been in the past recklessly forced on helpless schoolteachers, and in educational meetings the blackboards were at one time filled with drawings of ganglion cells and tables of reaction times. No warning against such "yellow psychology" can be serious enough.

The lawyer and the judge and the jurymen are sure that they do not need the experimental psychologists…they go on thinking that their legal instinct and their common sense supplies them with all that is needed and somewhat more; and if the time is ever to come when even the jurist is to show some concession to the spirit of modern psychology, public opinion will have to exert some pressure.

There has been an automobile accident. The one witness said that the automobile was running very slowly; the other, that he had never seen an automobile rushing more rapidly…the other day to most reliable expert shorthand writer's felt sure they had heard the utterances which they wrote down, and yet the records differed widely in important points.

Thus there remained the unintentional mistakes of the sound mind, and the psychologist must ask at once are they all of the same order.

The perception may be correct; its later reproduction may be false.

Is the court sufficiently aware of the great differences between men's perceptions and does the court take sufficient trouble to examine the capacities and habits with which the witness moves through the world which he believes he observes?

The demand that the memory of the witness should be tested with the methods of modern psychology has been raised sometimes, but it seems necessary to add that the study of his perceptive judgment will have to find its way into the court room too.

Of course, each study would be one-sided if the psychologist were only to emphasize the varieties of men and the differences by which one man's judgment and observation may be counted on to throw out an opposite report from that of another man. No, the psychologist in the courtroom should certainly have given not less attention to the analysis of these delusions. The jurymen and the judge do not discriminate whether the witness tells what he saw in late twilight—a woman in a red gown or one in a blue gown they are not expected to know that such a faint light would still allow the blue-collar sensation to come in, while the red color sensation would have disappeared.

Not every sworn statement is accepted as absolute reality. Contradictions between witnesses are too familiar. But the instinctive doubt refers primarily to veracity. The public in the main suspects that the witness lies, while taking for granted that if he is normal and conscious of responsibility he may forget a thing, but it would not believe that he could remember the wrong thing. The confidence in the reliability of memory is so general that the suspicion of memory illusions eventually plays a small role in the mind of the jurymen, and even the cross-examining lawyer is mostly dominated by the idea that a false statement is the product of intentional falsehood. All this is a popular illusion against which modern psychology must seriously protest.... no jurymen would be expected to follow his general impressions in the question as to whether the blood on a murderer's shirt is human or animal. But he is expected to make up his mind as to whether the memory ideas of a witness conflict with our objective reproductions of earlier experience or are mixed up with associations and suggestions.

It is so much easier everywhere to be satisfied with sharp demarcation lines and to listen only to a yes or a no; the man is sane or insane, and if he is saying, he speaks the truth or he lies. The psychologist would upset the satisfaction completely.

We may try hard to think of a name and it will not appear in consciousness; and when we have thought of something else for a long time, the desired name suddenly slips into our mind may it not be in a similar way that the effort for correct recollection under oath may prove powerless to a degree which public opinion under estimates? And no subjective feeling of certainty can be an objective criterion for the desired truth.

In the life of justice trains are wrecked and ships are colliding too often, simply because the law does not care to examine the mental color blindness of the witnesses' memory. And yet we have not even touched one factor which, more than anything else, devastates memory and plays havoc with our best intended recollections: that is, the power of suggestion.

Man has the power to hide his knowledge and his memories by silence and by lies and the infliction of physical and mental pain has always seemed the quickest way to untie the tongue and force the confession of truth.... under pain and fear a man may make any admission which will relieve his suffering, and, still more misleading, his mind may lose the power to discriminate between illusion and memory... [the psychologist] makes visible that which remains otherwise invisible, and shows any new facts which allow a clear diagnosis.

The study of the association of ideas has attracted students of the human mind since the day of Aristotle... associationists have begun to explain our entire mental life as essentially the interplay of such associations.

For instance, our purpose may be to find out whether a suspected person has really participated in a certain crime. He declares that he is innocent, that he was not present when the outrage occurred, and that he is not even familiar with the locality. An innocent man will not object to our proposing a series of 100 associations to demonstrate his innocence. A guilty man, of course, will not object, either, as a declination would indicate a fear of betraying himself; he cannot refuse and yet affirm his innocence. Moreover, he will feel sure that no questions can bring out any facts he wants to keep hidden in his soul; he will be on the lookout.... the suspected person may have self-control enough not to give away the dangerous idea directly; but the suppressed idea remains in consciousness, contains the next association, without his knowledge.

The first problem for the psychologist was whether the confession of a witness was a chain of conscious lies or whether he himself really believed what he told the court.

The "third-degree" may brutalize the mind and force either correct or falsified secrets to light..

CHAPTER FIVE

Lying and Truth

A man is measured by the angle at which he looks at objects.
~Ralph Waldo Emerson~

Lying

Lying is considered one of the great sins. Lying is the deliberate choice not to provide full and accurate information. Indeed, the Bible clearly declares, "keep thee far from a false matter" (Exodus 23:7). Leviticus 19:11 says, "thou shall not steal, thou shall not deny falsely, and thou shalt not lie to one another." Exodus 20:16 states, "thou shalt not bear false witness," which appears to apply to witnesses in court. Leviticus 19:36 states, "you shall have just scales, just weights, a just dry measure, and a just liquid measure," which refers to proper business interactions.

Controversy exists over the permissibility of the innocuous lie, known as the "little white lie." Lying for the purpose of causing pain or anguish in another person is prohibited. Commonplace are the occasions when one lies and no one suffers, or they suffer less. Lying undertaken for a laudable purpose, such as to prevent causing a person distress, is considered permissible. Lying for the purpose of preserving or prolonging life is sanctioned and not considered a transgression. But lying, even to reduce stress in a sick person, assumes that the recipient of the lie would agree to being lied to. Since the innocuous lie is sanctioned, some fear that it will cause the recipient distress.

There is still a greater risk, though, that the recipient will ultimately discover the truth and this will cause even greater harm than would have occurred if the full disclosure had been revealed from the onset. Lies have been distinguished as those which are *injurious, officious or jocose*. A jocose lie is told for entertainment and amusement. An officious lie is also known as a white lie—not intended to cause any harm; it is a lie of excuse and contrived to benefit somebody. An injurious lie has malicious, self-serving or harmful intent.

An interesting debate comes from the use of deception in clinical studies involving placebos. The investigator intentionally deceives the research subject about the placebo. It is a lie. Of course, the subject expects the placebo risk; otherwise they could never consent to the study. The problem, though, is that research would like to see no response to the placebo and a robust response to the active treatment. If subjects exposed to the placebo report a response from a sham treatment, they are, in fact, responding positively to a deception. The question is: why would someone feel a real and positive response to a lie? This is called *response expectancy*.[51] Ethical concerns exist about lying to patients, and although the deception is somewhat similar to a "white lie," the research lie is not to help the patient as much as it is to help the researcher prove a point. The positive placebo responder, who feels the absence of anxiety, is telling the truth about how he feels, but the cause of that reduced anxiety is unrelated to the altered factors. The placebo responder ought not to feel better. Is the patient lying to himself and the researcher? This is not malingering because it is the patient's *bona fide* feeling. A positive response to a placebo means that some other, perhaps unknown, mechanism is producing the end result. The response, unrelated to the treatment, is very real to the patient. The question is—what psychological aspects of the placebo responder produced the response? Does the deception bring to the relationship an acquiescence that the patient can, in turn, deceive the researchers? The patient knows he may have been tested with a deception. Might he doubt his own feelings? Indeed, what effect will it have on the person's psychology if they learn they did respond to a deception? And can this person be used in future studies if they are known to positively respond to deception? Placebo use could help identify malingers. I would expect that a non-malingering placebo responder will feel amazement, and perhaps some shame at being so gullible. A malingering placebo responder would not be at all surprised that he was given a placebo, and would feel dim-witted and angry that he was caught.

This thought can be extended to the process of testing for malingering and deception. The sophisticated criminal knows the test questions are being used to trick him into a series of responses that will unmask the truth. The unsophisticated criminal, or the mentally retarded or impaired criminal, may not consider the test to have a "trick" quality. In either case, the interviewer often approaches the subject with this type of common verbiage: "I would like to ask you a series of questions so we can learn more about you..."

The doctor, however, is really saying, "I am giving you a set of anchor points which will let me know if you are lying."

The malingering subject thinks, "Can I figure out the test question patterns so my lie is not discovered?"

What happens when researchers feel comfort in maintaining a "lie" to arrive at the truth? This is a major ethical concern because such a routine can corrupt the professionals who practice it. The practice might also grow into a larger personal disposition that deception is permitted in the name of a goal. This is especially so when professionals and authorities willingly employ the technique; this has resulted in this statement in the American Psychological Association's guidelines for research.

The APA Guideline 8.07[52] states: "(a) psychologists do not conduct a study involving deception unless they have determined that the use of deceptive techniques is justified by the study's significant prospective scientific, education or applied value and that effective nondeceptive alternative procedures are not feasible; (b) psychologists do not deceive prospective participants about the research that is reasonably expected to cause physical pain or severe emotional distress; (c) psychologists explain any deception that is an integral feature of the design and conduct of an experiment to participants as early as feasible, preferably at the conclusion of their participation, but no later than at the conclusion of the data collection, and permit participants to withdraw their data."

One very savvy criminal defendant told me he never trusted prosecution-hired psychologists who were sent to examine him—he saw them as agents of the prosecutor, and if he felt the state attorney was twisting and lying about facts of the case, then the psychologist was "merely one of their puppets…I've been examined too many times, and I can see the patterns in the questions…they also don't be as friendly, it's like too mechanical and they don't want to know a lot about me outside of the tests…give me a defense psychologist, and they are friendlier and a lot more comfortable to talk to. They actually scare me more, 'cause I sometimes let my guard down about the real me." This is a classic example of the halo effect.

Many times the subject does not hear about the deceptive techniques used until, in court, they hear opposing counsel's experts criticize the test, techniques and results.

Is deception necessary to test for deception? Often—yes. What effect does a court order have on testing trustworthiness—is the subject's willingness to assent to the process a significant variable? In a sense, court orders to test for malingering using tests are a form of authorized deception. If the evaluator did not explicitly tell the subject that he is being examined to test for malingering—e.g., "I am now going to use a test designed to see if you are lying or not," then a violation of consent to testing may exist. What requirement exists to reveal the purpose and design of a test before it is used? Is the process akin to a search warrant?

The testing process can become an entertaining bout of wits and cleverness—a first-class evaluator can be seriously challenged by a first-rate liar.

It has been said that those who give officious lies should gulp the lie the same as a person who takes distasteful but necessary medicine.

I heard that "Lying has also been considered the product of the intentional negation of subjective truth." (I cannot find the source.) This suggests that a prerequisite of deception is the inhibition of truth. St. Thomas Aquinas defined lying as a "statement at variance with the mind." This indicates that some forethought exists in the planning and before the presentation of a statement that is knowingly contrary to the truth. Theologians often define lying as a statement that is the opposite of truth. Truth is a correspondence between what is being claimed and the objective veracity of that claim. That is, truth exists when different people have the same interpretation and find the same significance in the item or event that is being evaluated. In other words, the manifestation—in our case, the claimed psychiatric symptoms—must be consistent with a real presence of psychopathology. Although there are many evolving elements to the science and definitions of psychiatric illnesses, hopefully, it is more concrete then the issues debated within ethics and religion. No absolute truth exists insofar as the full scope of religion and ethics is concerned, but there is hope that greater objective "truths" are evolving in the developments of making a psychiatric diagnosis. A real problem exists because we dvo not have irrefutable and absolutely accurate diagnostic tools.

There is also a sense in our society that each person will have such self-regard and self-dignity that they will not engage in lies.

A person who claims an allegiance and commitment to a social order, but who lies, would be considered a hypocrite. Hypocrites cannot be trusted to be honest and this loss of confidence produces an injury to the entire community. Being hypocritical is not a harmless event. It violates the expectation of truth, which becomes a detriment to others. And it can also try to serve the purpose of avoiding responsibility for an action.

Everyday life challenges those who possess integrity. For example: People often praise a bride for her beauty. But what to do if she is decidedly not beautiful?[53] Silence may be the most appropriate response, otherwise a very diplomatic response needs to be crafted that is instructive, honest, but not destructive to the bride and her community. Too often, falsehoods are allowed to live under a cloak that hides a painful reality, and if that cloak is obvious to many in our community, it could rise to level of acceptance as normal and customary. To an objective observer, this is collective hypocrisy.

There is also a common consensus that no obligation to disclose the truth exists if the recipient is not entitled to the information. For example, St. Augustine, who felt that the truth must be told at all times, offers a case in which murderers are looking for a man. The intended victim is hiding in your house. If the murderers come and ask where this intended victim is, you can say that you know where he is, but will not tell.

Police are commonly given wide latitude in deceiving suspects in order to ferret out the truth.

Many people believe that it is perfectly permissible to deceive an enemy. If a statesman or a doctor is asked questions about which he cannot talk without breaching a confidence or trust, then the correct answer is that he has no "communicable" knowledge.

Uttering a general lie is commonly considered intrinsically wrong, and yet the question so perplexing is that if it is lawful to kill for one's own self-defense, might it at times be lawful to tell a lie in one's own self-defense?

The customary belief is that those who utter consciously-made false statements are not permitted to escape responsibility.

Aristotle felt people should never lie, but Plato felt that physicians can lie to patients when it is for their own good. A statesman can lie to the public when it is for a greater welfare. Augustine proposed a hierarchy of eight types of lies ranging from falsehoods in the "religious doctrine" to lies that do not hurt anybody. Many modern thinkers fall into two camps: those who absolutely shun lying regardless of the costs, and those who believe that prevarication is sometimes necessary and even permissible.

Lying in order to benefit others is often permitted. Malingering is typically lying to benefit oneself. Malingering to save one's life, such as being too sick to work in a prisoner of war camp is motivationally and ethically different than the typical malingering situation. This is quite obvious.

If someone is lying to achieve a wicked intention, then he is denying the recipient of his deception the right to hear the truth. If the person who hears the lie is charged with the responsibility of making a social or judicial decision based on the information given him, then he might clearly perpetuate the lie, which would serve not the greater good, but only the individual needs of the original liar. Two social violations occur here. First is the lying for one's own needs, and the second is disrespect for the effects of the decision-making process.

That being said, the obligation exists to extract an understanding of how lying, as a survival technique, develops in a suspected malingerer. This requires a thorough exploration of the experiential and psychodynamic history of the person's life. While it may not necessarily excuse the person from any liability for his actions, it explains how the situation arose. It also shines valuable light on potential rehabilitation because it identifies the real motivations. Too often we punish for the acts and ignore the powerful motivations behind the acts. It is not enough, and it distracts from civilized sophistication and moral development, if we simply call a person a "liar" without attaching the information as to why the person lied. Indeed, Bok feels that we should see if a lie is justifiable and that one aspect of that test would be to look at our own conscience and ask how we would act if the roles and experiences in life had been reversed.[54]

Truth

Lying has been discussed, so the concept of truth must also be examined.

Truth is the process whereby people share their knowledge and experiences with honesty and integrity. There should be no contradictions in the scope, factual basis of, or response to truth between those who give the information and those who receive it. Yet those declaring the 'truth' regularly infuse their declarations with their own flavors, perfumes and margins. Those who offer truth must try to painfully test their conclusions for syllogistic flaws or biases.

Evaluating someone who is psychotic is almost always done by someone who has never been psychotic. The same cannot be said for malingering. Examiners who have the mindset to malinger might better identify malingering. Likewise, examiners who are less inclined to malinger might be less skillful at identifying malingers. Serious questions emerge in what might be accepted as boundaries of truth.

In summary, the examiner with the stronger personal disposition to malinger may report malingering more freely than otherwise might be the case. Over-reporting malingering is a risk. There may also be a tendency not to identify the type of or the real reasons for the malingering. He acts like a local meteorologist. The examiner with a stronger personal posture not to malinger may report less frequent malingering because he is identifies with other aspects of the person's history—he is the global meteorologist.

Merriam-Webster's word of the year was the term that was looked up the most on m-w.com, but this year, the dictionary publisher opened up the choice to the public in an online vote. The word selected by a five to one margin was truthiness, *which was the American Dialect Society's pick for WOTY in 2005. 'Truthiness' was coined by Stephen Colbert on his television show The Colbert Report in October 2005. (There are a handful of earlier uses, but Colbert probably independently coined it and his use of the term is the root of its current popularity.) Truthiness was defined by Colbert as: "truth that comes from the gut, not books." The American Dialect Society gave it a more lexicographic treatment by defining it as: the quality of preferring concepts or facts one wishes to be true, rather than concepts or facts known to be true.* [55]

One of the theories of truth is known as the "coherence theory of truth." The classic example is the statement "snow is white and cold." This fact is considered true if the statement from the speaker is coherent with the experience of the listener. Truth is defined as the effect that a fact has on us and that this effect is in agreement with reality and is accepted as a common sensation among people. Truth produces an emotional bond and a sense of familiarity between the speaker and the listener. This may be the physiological result of mirror neurons.

The mathematician seeks truth that should apply throughout the universe. The same goes for the scientists. But the accepted level of truth for the justice or the ethicist is based on a much more regional set of values—these are far more likely to be opinions that have been given the status of a law. This is in an interesting contrast to the Ten Commandments, which are essentially God-given laws and not human opinions. Believers will interpret the God-given laws to have much more universality than those which are human opinions that have been converted into laws. Yet, if someone is in the legal system, a punishment for an action will be based on a law, which is assumed to be a truth, but that truth may actually be a local opinion and not universal truth.

If something is true, then there is no "more or less" quality to it.

CHAPTER SIX

Testing of malingering — The Diagnostic Process

I asked a prisoner if anyone in the world would really know if he was lying or being honest. He said, "Ask my Momma—I can't do nothing she don't catch…"

Because legal or financial ramifications rest on the accurate diagnosis of malingering, the diagnostic process needs to envelop as full a gamut as possible of the variables causing human behavior. Mere observations can be deceptive. In fact, even the observers must disclose themselves as a variable on the list of diagnostic anchor and bias points.[56] Like the prisoner who told me to talk to his "Momma," one major obstacle against a trustworthy diagnosis is that our databases are too limited. His "Momma" could reliably read and convert his nuances so as to understand a particular behavior. That depth of data usually does not exist with most professional evaluators. A skilled malingerer intentionally tries to hide such nuances.

Is it possible to utilize the tools used to diagnose malingering to predict it as well? As science evolves, the ethical use of such skills can cause problems. This is relevant to the new debate with regards to genetic testing—will people with specific genetic patterns find it impossible to be insured? Should they be allowed to procreate? What role will we assign them in a society if we know that their genetic makeup will cause disease or other problems?

It would not be inconceivable to envision a new caste system. This is known as the problem of prediction. Will our scientific knowledge allow us to make predictions about a person's future? If we know someone has a genetic predisposition to malinger, will they be permitted to rise to positions of social authority?

Great constraint is mandatory here because there exists no perfect means of prediction. Scientific knowledge is much too limited to make predictions based on "soft" science associations (sometimes known as "junk science" or pseudoscience), beliefs and opinions. Powerful statistical associations may themselves not demonstrate true scientific cause-and-effects, yet, for example, a criminal situation may see courts choose to act on the side of precaution, which is understandable given their mandate to protect society. But the "diagnosis" may still be wrong.

Predictions are often inaccurate because the scientific basis behind the particular test was wrong for the situation, because the test was poorly performed, or because the test was done with a bias. But imagine how appetizing—and therefore how mesmeric it would be to society, if someone offered a unfussy instrument that would also be a guaranteed predictor of future violence, sexual abuse, stealing, et cetera?

Courts need to correctly distinguish between the relatively less dangerous, typical non-recidivist criminal from the truly dangerous and recidivistic one. Part of that process demands knowledge about the presence of an uncontrollable psychiatric condition or propensity. This knowledge helps predict if a danger exists because the criminal cannot be rehabilitated. The court must raise these questions: (1) can the pathology causing the criminal behavior be corrected with current methodologies, and (2) if treatment is scientifically available, is it also truly available with the degree of consistency, sophistication, and intensity needed to rehabilitate the criminal? If the treatment levels needed to rehabilitate the criminal are not available, then the court may have to consider incarceration or long-term hospitalization in order to protect society. Many malingers require such a degree and sophistication of treatment that effective treatment is not possible. The problem lies, however, in the frequent misdiagnosis of malingering stemming from sloppy or biased examiners.

Numerous rating scales assist to make the diagnostic process objective, but they actually only help to identify some of the more obvious characteristics of malingering. Detailed psychosocial and psychiatric histories also help, but the examiner should be wary if they are based primarily on chart reviews, which report only potentially soiled data; they carry the limitations and partiality of the various contributors to the charts. A typical chart explores little more than nursing-level behavioral observations or mental status examinations. Scant in-depth detail about the subject's biopsychosocial background is more common than not. Mention may be made of traumas, but often without any detailed investigations into the full impact of these events. A psychodynamic explanation is a rare diagnostic treasure.

Experts disagree because they use or differ in how they value various data points. One would hope that all the experts would come to the same conclusion. A diagnosis should not be a matter of opinion, but of fact. When experts disagree, there may be a number of causes. It may be because either the diagnostic entity itself is insufficiently defined, or that the sense of a cluster is invariant of the diagnostic entity (which again speaks to problems in the primary definition of the diagnosis or limitations in the specificity and reliability of the diagnostic tools). Another cause of dissension might arise from the experts interpreting data either with unequal levels of skill and/or with biases.

Malingering is a product of data presentation and data interpretation by both the patient and the examiner. Understanding motivation is a time- and investigatory-intensive process. The first step is to both assume that the person is not malingering and that the examiner is objectively skilled and impartial.

Then the medical/psychiatric condition needs to be treated unless the symptoms are blatantly unrealistic. If psychoses are claimed, then treatment must follow. Interventions must be sufficient so that long-term behavioral changes can occur and can be repeatedly observed. Careful and sophisticated clinical investigations are mandatory. These include detailed biopsychosocial histories, consideration of offensive versus a defensive malingering, a study of the person's ego structure and relationship to shame, and an in-depth record of real didactic interactions over time, which test the analytic suppositions.

The presence or intensity of psychoses or other aberrant behaviors may fluctuate, and these shifts cannot be assumed to suggest malingering or manipulative behaviors. Some of it may be situational as well. For example, someone with a severe obsessive-compulsive disorder may become intolerant and argumentative if not allowed to reduce an obsession or a compulsion. Staff may mistakenly see this as "once he got his way, he calmed down." Likewise, those suffering borderline personality disorders may have transient psychotic episodes or mood swings that are merely responding to environmental changes.

When psychoses are claimed, it is helpful to look at the presence of positive versus negative symptoms as a test for malingering. Malingering will more likely present with the positive rather than the negative symptoms.

A full diagnostic workup for a thought disorder should include:

- *Look for the positive and negative symptoms associated with the proffered condition.*
- *Consider the prior treatment history of the similar symptoms. Were the treatments adequate and aggressive enough? Perhaps they need to be retested. A failure to respond may be an inaccurate diagnosis or reflect inadequate or unavailable treatment. Study failed treatments. Failed treatments are not automatically indicative of malingering. Get clinical and historical data from family, co-workers and friends.*
- *Explore for typical co-morbidities, including medical or neurological disorders, exposure to toxins, perinatal problems, et cetera. Seek anchor points in a person's life. Establish periods when things were good and when things were bad. Explore why these differences occurred. Look carefully at the onset of the alleged symptoms. That a person*

did not have symptoms before the start of criminal activity does not
necessarily disconnect them from a disease involvement that may have
legitimately started concurrently.

- *Determine the time course of dysfunction. Was the person functioning*
  well before the event which is now explained by the alleged
  malingering?
- *Keep every diagnosis as a hypothesis as long as possible. The imperative*
  test is to treat the proffered condition, capture new data during the
  treatment process, and suitably report the outcome.

Frequently there is neither the time nor the money available
to do all the above.

The hypothesis is often made that the person "learned to be
psychotic" from fellow inmates or other sources. If this is suspected,
then it is important to know how the person felt and acted before
he was arrested, when the symptoms started, his understanding
of the etiology of the symptoms, does he know other people with
similar symptoms, what his mood was like before the symptoms
started, and what he has heard that will make the symptoms go
away? It may quite difficult to get this information.

It is also important to ask or explore how the patient responds
when people lie to him.

An inmate, charged with carjacking, claimed hallucinations
told him to steal the car. There was no history of drug abuse or prior
psychiatric issues. He told the jail nurse about his hallucinations;
he was assigned to the psychiatric unit. In my interview, I told
them that some people might accuse him of lying about the

hallucinations. I also told him that they would be looking at him very closely and would probably also speak to his friends and family, as well as look for any prior medical records. I told them that my job was to try to get a real picture of what was going on with him, but that he needed to know that there were other things that may be brought to court other than what he tells me.

He said, "you mean they think I'm lying?"

I said, "Yes."

That initiated a general discussion about how people respond when they have been lied to, and I followed this with questions about how he felt if he learned that he had been lied to, especially on important issues. As we spoke, and I questioned him more in a therapeutic fashion as opposed to an interrogatory one, I saw more disbelief than nervousness. A timorous, almost bashful quality emerged. He was clearly not as hostile. Ultimately he told me that the hallucinations have been present for quite some time, but he was embarrassed to tell anyone about them, and that after a breakup with his girlfriend, the hallucinations finally got so out of control that he could not resist them. He stole the car and then was arrested. He could not explain why he found the inner strength to tell the nurse about the hallucinations other than the fact that he was mature enough now to recognize how much trouble he was in. He could not hide any longer because the social shame and humiliation of having a psychosis was less than the fright of being in jail.

Another case highlights the opposite response to the questions about how someone responds to being lied to. A nineteen-year-old woman with a series of arrests for petty crimes and drug abuse insisted that she went into this lifestyle after a childhood of multiple emotional and physical abuses. In the course of the interview, it became evident that she handled her considerable psychological discomfort in life with denial and an energetic manipulation of her world to keep her pain at bay. She would clearly play one person against the other, very much in the style of a borderline personality disorder. Often this would require fabrications and prevarications. She also admitted that it was intolerable to her when people were not honest or truthful—that made her angry. We were later able to ascertain that dishonesty in others frightened her. So, when I challenged her with the fact that other people involved in the case may consider her claims of being out of control related to her lifetime of traumas as being a "convenient effort to explain away her criminal activity," she became annoyed. She was being "challenged." She did not like that, and, while psychodynamically her core pathology was probably very valid and very real, and her ego was probably extremely frail, it was evident that she was definitely over-dramatizing her psychopathology in order to control the situation. But this was her character style, and this character grew out of her experiences and lack of other skills. Nonetheless, her chosen behaviors were more offensive. There was also a component in her reports that did not avail itself to a real test of the report's validity. Clearly very narcissistic qualities existed. She also said to me, "that other doctor, he came here and asked questions, and we didn't talk like this, you know, calm and slow, and some of them questions were kinda odd, and I asked why he asked those questions, and I kinda got not to trust him, so maybe I wasn't so honest with him..."

To be true to malingering, the malingerer must elevate the sophistication of reported symptoms in advance and in response to the examiner's increasing the level of testing points about the reported symptoms. This symptom rise leads to clinical examination step-ups—the doctor should ask new questions which the patient may not know how to answer. The patient then offers new data which he wants the doctor to accept. The diagnostic testing usually ends when the doctor is no longer able to validate symptoms. This is harder to do with psychiatric than physical symptoms. For example, few patients know about dermatomes, so questions about symptoms that follow dermatome distributions may be an excellent field on which to test for feigning.

One interview technique is to surprise the suspected malingerer with a comment such as, "commonly, people with your symptoms also have the sensation of changes over their body. Do you have any strange sensations or lack of feeling, weakness, anywhere on your body?" This is, of course, an opportunity to embellish feigned symptoms and to add to the patient's list of complaints about responses that cannot be feigned. Experienced and sophisticated patients taunt the process. A patient who succeeds can humiliate the examiner. The goal is to surreptitiously and diplomatically challenge the patient with as much non-feignable data as possible.

Merely observing a patient can be misleading. People need to survive and so interact accordingly to their environment. That someone may have some social interactions with other inmates does not preclude significant psychopathology. Believing that laughing, sitting and playing cards, or helping to serve food in a jail cell to win extra recreation time qualifies to discount the presence of real psychopathology is dangerously presumptuous.

A twenty-two-year-old was charged with murder. He was also significantly mentally retarded. The state alleged he was exaggerating his retardation. A deputy testified that he saw the defendant playing Monopoly, and the state used this observation to suggest he was malingering. In fact, however, the defendant did not understand the game and was merely playing *with* the Monopoly game. "I liked to roll the dice and buy things..." He did not appreciate that the game was to accumulate real estate and get rent from the other players.

Asking the patient how they would react to the possibility that their claimed illness will never get better, or perhaps worsen over time, can often elicit interesting commentary about the person's self-perceived future. Essentially, the question asks what it was that made them ill and what do they think might make them better. If the answers are too simplistic and glib, then malingering may exist. How a suspected malingerer responds to an offer of a prolonged and intense hospitalization is extremely revealing about their comfort level with their chosen set of presented symptoms. There is no fear or hesitancy with genuine symptoms because no acting exists. If they are not genuine, a great deal of energy would have to be devoted to ensuring symptom consistency over time. Sophisticated notes of behavior, interactions, moods and motivations, along with repeated testing over time and under different conditions, would produce a rich objective biography. Such a test produces a measure of comfort versus discomfort in the patient. Those who feign will have to study how to expand the sick role.

CHAPTER SEVEN

Professionals who find—
And those who do not find—malingering

Draftsmen can be trained. Colorists are born.
~Litten~

There are few things that rattle me more than when another mental health evaluator's impression of a patient is the opposite of mine. I run to my database, fearing I may have overlooked some key item.

One clear distinction is that the evaluations may occur at different times, so the existing clinical picture might be different. The other essential difference is that all examiners are not equally skilled. Each may not weigh the same data in a similar manner. These points may help explain the dissimilar results:

Medication use—did the separate evaluations occur before or after medications were started?

A bipolar patient committed a crime after he stopped his medications. The initial jail evaluations reported grandiosity and denial, and that he said he was healthy and innocent. Six weeks of medication changed his mental status and he accepted that he had stolen the car.

While in a forensic hospital a 22 year old male was given three psychiatric medications. A in-hospital evaluation occurred while taking these medications and the examiner declared him to be competent. I later examined him in the local jail after two of these medications had been stopped. I reported what I observed and felt he was incompetent.

Are there any medical problems being addressed, or not addressed, that impact a mental status?

A seventy-eight year-old diabetic was not given enough insulin for the two weeks in jail. I saw him when his blood sugars were normal. The first examiner saw him shortly after his arrest when he suffered both the separation from his medications and the effect that stress can have on glycemic control.

A young man murder his girlfriend. Part of his agitation stemmed from his thyroid toxicosis. A non-medically trained examiner did not consider this matter.

A 50 year old was charged with embezzling. It was uncharacteristic of him. Eventually a neurologist found a unexpected frontal lobe dysfunction, but a psychologist did not believe this was sufficient evidence to exclude malingering.

How long has the person been incarcerated? Someone newly-jailed, or incarcerated for the first time may have a different response to the legal system than one who has been waiting in jail for over a year. People change psychologically when in jail for long periods of time. Their approach to their situation may subsequently change.

"I be here a long time. I thought I be able to handle it. Now I wanna get it over. I miss my kids…listen, let me tell you what really happened…"

A hearing impaired elderly man convicted of murder was awaiting trial on additional charges. He was kept in solitary confinement for over a year with very little sensory stimulation. He hallucinated voices at night and complained of the Gestapo. Eventually he revealed to me how as a 10 year French Jew his family escaped after Germans' tortured his friends and family.

Did the other examiner have additional data not given to me?

The prosecutor did not give the public defender certain telltale domestic violence and business records. Yet, at the time of our respective examinations, the state's expert had those records. I did not. The state examiner did not tell the defendant that he had those records. The defendant lied to me, saying no prior sticky history existed. I reminded the defendant that lying about past activities was dangerous because someone might later find something. He insisted nothing would be found. At the time of my examination, I used my database to make my initial opinion.

Between the evaluations, was the patient moved into a different unit in the jail? Real differences exist between general population cells, psychiatric units, life-skill or drug-treatment units, etc. Sometimes prisoners will feign to get into a better unit, and once there, the intensity of the lying may change.

A young boy repeatedly engaged in minor thefts. He was initially cocky and defiant. But he was also very mad at his estranged father and his weak mother. His initial response to incarceration was defiance. Fortunately he was moved to a juvenile life-skills unit where he received excellent counseling. The initial stubborn insistence that "I am alright" changed to a more insightful "...okay, thanks, I'm better now...I gotta figure out what is really me..."

A very anxious young man was moved to a psychiatric unit where, in time, he taught other inmates to sketch. He felt a purpose in life, received accolades and decided to seek graphic arts training. His behavior in general population had been defiant and hostile. Doctors thought he was faking the anxiety but offered treatment. The anxiety did not exist in the psychiatric unit.

Has the patient been getting counseling or family visits? If not incarcerated, then what family support, counseling or other changes have occurred since the arrest?

"That lady minister keeps coming here...you know, she makes sense. I see what I gotta do now."

"My wife had her sister tell me she's filing for a divorce. Doesn't she know how sick she's making me? I get rashes—here, look, look at my chest. I don't know, I don't know....she made this all happen, and now she's making it worse, and me being in jail.... I hope she's real happy now..."

Have the charges been changed? Does the person feel wrongly accused?

"They dropped the burglary charge but said I raped her. I never raped her! Yeh, all this came down yesterday. I could spit in the cop's face. Am I sick, you're damned right I am, and you going pay for this. My blood pressure is way up, the doc here won't see me until next week, I know I'm going have a stroke, it'll be your fault if I die, I need medical help, man. I need it now!"

Sometimes prisoners know themselves very well. Many of them do indeed have various intensities of psychopathology.

One prisoner knew he could not sleep in the general population, which would eventually lead to a depression, so he feigned depression, which got him into a psychiatric unit. He was given antidepressant treatment, and he felt safe and could sleep.

Does the patient have a personality style or disorder which presents in a gruff or demanding way? Perhaps the other evaluator could not couple with the patient in such a way that a non-contentious interview could ensue.

An attractive eighteen-year-old girl was arrested for battery on an officer. She had been the victim of repeated sexual abuse. A male guard punished her for speaking out of turn. She was furious at him and was still so at the time of our meeting. She kept telling me that there was nothing wrong with her that other people did not cause. I returned for a second visit after she'd been moved to a life-skills unit. The therapy helped her accept her contributions to her troubles.

How long did the individual evaluators spend with the patient?

"The one doc spent a long time but he only gave me tests and we did a little talking. Another doc only asked questions and we spoke a lot about my family—I don't know how long he was with me, but it was shorter than the first guy, but I know I said more…then a third guy came in and he was in and out like a scared rabbit—I took a test and it felt like he was gone."

A time sheet of symptoms is critical, but it is not always available. So answers to these questions are usually sewn together from scattered pieces. As a result, differing professional opinions come from (1) the extrapolation formula each examiner used to fill in the missing pieces, or (2) the number of data points available to the rater.

A kernel of truth in the data may suggest malingering. That kernel can frighten the court, suggesting that more malingering really exists but has not yet been found. The "malingering diagnosis" is one of extrapolation and probability. Acting on it offers social comfort more than justice.

"The person might be dangerous, so let's be conservative" is the subtle recommendation to the court. A thorough examiner must test the "menacing" kernel and try to expand it into a diagnosis with prognostic abilities. Elsewhere in the book is a discussion of the difference between qualitative and quantitative data analysis. Is the malingering diagnosis a qualitative analysis clothed in only the style of a quantitative outfit?

Can experts differ and still be experts? Obviously one expert is right and the other is wrong.

The news talk shows intrigue me. So too do the stock market watchers. There is no consensus, they argue based on their opinions of events and data, they all have different solutions to common problems, they interpret history differently, and they attest to their solutions with a conviction of proven fact and not theory. When an event finally happens, such as an election, these same people return to explain why their original mantras failed or were successfully predictive. Here are a few related thoughts:

"A great many people think they are thinking when they are merely rearranging their prejudices."—*William James*

"Most people educate their prejudices…" —*Josh Billings, 1874*

"The best reformers the world has ever seen are those who commence on themselves."—*George Bernard Shaw, 1949*

"There are as many opinions as there are experts."—*Franklin D. Roosevelt, 1942*

"For the great enemy of the truth is very often not the lie—deliberate, contrived, and dishonest—but the myth—persistent, persuasive, and unrealistic. Too often we hold fast to the clichés of our forbearers. We subject all facts to prefabricated sets of interpretations. We enjoy the comfort of opinion without the discomfort of thought." —*J.F. Kennedy, 1962*

Clearly one of the problems rests on the ability to identify sufficient quantities of objective data such that when given to anyone, they will all be forced—by the consistent nature of the data—to come to the same conclusions.

An expert is actually a witness to a test. These professional, but nonetheless, personal observations are reported to a court or authority. Expert witnesses do not see the offense, so, unlike fact witnesses, they offer opinions based on a retrospective review of what other people saw and reported. They prepare a projection-based opinion on the mental status at the time of an event in the past. If asked, they also perform a diagnostic examination on a current mental status, and obviously a functional current mental status is needed for a constructive interview to occur.

Retrospective analysis incorporates all prior analytical biases or errors to enter into the new opinion. After all, it would be expected that two experts, with similar databases, ought to arrive at very similar opinions. Eyewitnesses are also not above error—memory lapses, confusion, or other situations may reduce the trustworthiness of their reports. And though one hopes it may not be, an eyewitness can also infuse their reports with their own biases—it is not impossible for the eyewitness to color their facts with some opinion. Police reports are generally good summaries, but a report is a limited gathering of all facts and influences—it, too, may have a bias towards an opinion as well by virtue of what is omitted (or unknown) about the situation.

A long-haul truck driver was hit by a recklessly speeding car. All passengers in that car died. The police entirely exonerated the truck driver, but a witness, and friend of the deceased, claimed the truck driver was using the cell phone and not paying attention to his driving. The family of the deceased therefore initiated a civil suit against the driver. The driver insisted he was not using the phone. Phone records showed no calls, but the witness said he may have been just starting to make a call.

Expert witnesses also opine on what they themselves see or measure. They are also not above weaving their own values into an opinion. After all, an expert's opinion is gauged as much by what is written in the report as what is not written in the report.

So how are experts and their opinions used in the court? A brief history will help. In 1923, James Frye was accused of murder. He wanted an expert to present data about the systolic blood pressure test. He felt the testimony would exonerate him from the crime. The judge denied the request because the science for that test had not achieved general acceptance in medicine. It was an early defense against fringe or junk science, and on the whole, the Frye ruling became the general standard test for scientific evidence until 1993.[57]

Daubert was born with abnormalities. In 1993, his parents sued Merrell Dow, claiming their drug, Bendectin,[58] caused birth defects. The actual association between the drug and birth defects was vigorously debated. A defense review of thirty safety studies of the drug failed to prove the connection. But the plaintiff asked eight other experts to present evidence to the contrary. The judge denied the plaintiff's request. Eventually the Supreme Court reversed the lower court's ruling.[59] The high court said the plaintiff's expert opinions could be entertained because they do not make the decision for the court, but rather provide data that would assist the trier of fact. Clinical diagnosing became the purview of the judge.

This is an interesting point insofar as malingering and lying is concerned. If psychological tests, examinations or the use of machine reports such as fMRI or brain mapping is used in court, then no question about lying exists because the data (when it is solidly proven) will make the data irrefutable.

Expert testimony can be introduced to help the jury reach a more informed judgment, but an expert's testimony cannot be the final determination of truth. This means that a jury could decide that the defendant is not lying even with scientific evidence to the contrary. If scientific data is not solidly established, then the jury could nullify the data and any expert's credibility. In fact, court testimony commonly focuses on one expert being used to discredit the other expert. Two opposing experts could nullify each other. It also makes diagnostic techniques look foolish, and this is especially so if they are costly, dressed in scientific language and mutually contradicting. This takes on the flavor of junk science.

The scientific debate can mock the diagnostic process. Each expert offers an opinion, the judge offers an opinion, and the jury opines as well. The final outcome is often a mixture of who made the most compelling or theatrically cohesive argument and what social or political implications exist behind one decision or another. An experienced trial attorney once told me there are really three possible outcomes to any case: guilty, not guilty and innocent.

Junk science is untested science that offers opinion as if it is equal to fact. A kernel of truth may exist in the junk science, or the thread with which it is stitched may appear to be scientific, but the final garment, as scientific sounding as it may be, just cloaks its proponents' beliefs or hopes.

Getting trustworthy data is a key concern in pharmaceutical research. They need to know if a medication is truly effective. Great effort is made to be certain that anyone who tests for the effect of a new medication is measuring a real effect. They also work very hard to reduce variances between raters. They want all raters, if presented with the same clinical presentation, to arrive at the same conclusion. The conclusion may not endorse their medication, but at least there is a *consistent* report from many independent raters. That gives trustworthiness to the final observations. Raters are now trained. They all study the same case, practice standardized rating scales, discuss differences they may have in their opinions about the case, compare their results with those of anonymous expert panels, and only then are they allowed to give opinions about real patients. These testing/refresher courses are repeated quite often, and a researcher might go through dozens of them in the course of their career.

Such examiner training does not happen in the court system. The usual questions are, "what is your training?...Have you been declared an expert before?" Junk science can walk right in! Using a panel of experts on a case ought to appreciably reduce this variability.

A brief primer on research will help illuminate the problem and guide us to a solution. A basic notion in research is to separate qualitative data from quantitative data. Basically, qualitative data is based on experience and intuition. Quantitative data is, in contrast, a statistical analysis of data. Qualitative data is "coded" before it is quantitatively analyzed, and the coding may be defective or biased. So any subsequent statistical analysis will produce imperfect observations. This is the mature and time-honored lesson of GIGO: "garbage in—garbage out," from the world of computer science.

This list may help explain the differences in data - and hypotheses - making and testing:

A qualitative analysis is often the precursor to a quantitative analysis. It is more the process of exploring or developing ideas. A quantitative analysis is more the process of testing the ideas. The differences are these:

Qualitative Analysis

- Develops theories
- Finds meanings in data or events
- A researcher's opinion can be part of the data
- Techniques are communication and observation
- Data collection is unstructured
- Multiple realties are used
- Bias might exist in the data collector
- Can accept non-numerical data
- Many events combine into a result
- Results may vary with time or place
- Create but not need to verify hypotheses

Quantitative Analysis

- Tests and develops theories
- Establishes relationships and causes
- A researcher's opinion is not part of the data
- Techniques use instruments and devices

- Data collection is structured
- A single reality is best
- Non bias in the data collector
- Requires numerical data
- Prefers one event leading to a result
- Believes its results can generalize or be universal
- Seeks to verify hypotheses

The beauty and scourge of the mental health profession is the "gut feeling." Even experienced clinicians may say that their impressions, i.e., their feelings, are being pulled in a certain direction. "Gut feelings" are often correct and may initially be contrary to the objective data in the file. This is because the "gut feeling" is, in reality, a sensitivity to nuances. Humans interact using countless overt, covert, loud and subtle clues. Clues are transmitted differently, based on the situations—a person who is frightened, in a rush, feeling ill, hallucinating or otherwise bothered will certainly give out different clues about themselves. The style and quality of revealed clues is a response to those around the person. A very formal, mechanical, rushed or tired examiner may miss, not pick up, or not even evoke clues. Examiners—themselves human—may be less sensitive to certain levels of clues. This might be a function of their mirror neurons.

In the mid-1990's it was discovered that the same group of neurons would discharge either when a monkey did an act or when it merely observed other monkey executing the same act. These were activities in what were called *mirror neurons*. Further study revealed that these same mirror responses occurred with just the sound of the action. This mirror neuron response was later found to exist in humans, with distinct regions in the premotor and posterior parietal cortices.

Through this mirroring process we become attuned to the intentional relations of others. It seems that this is a key process in explaining the mechanisms of understanding and empathy. By becoming attuned to "others," these "others" become more than a system, they become like us—"people." They become us. We simulate them as *us in us*. That simulation gives us a "common experience" from which we "understand" them. The "inexplicable gut feeling" we get from others may be an "unmediated resonance." The resonated feelings could be good, sad, tactile, painful, fearful, or any aspect of our experiences. At some level, these primary resonations may be immune from any cultural or social bias.

The basic simulation process may be a rudimentary brain function under no influence of will or conscious effort. We do not resonate on purpose, but the interaction does produce an outcome. The resonation is evaluated by psychological or cognitive data sets. A raw resonation gives us a sense of what the other person is feeling, and from that comes a picture of possible actions based on an inventory of, and processing biases, from prior experiences.

We tend to unconsciously resonate with others. Sometimes we try to resonate with others or want them to resonate with us. We may feel a resonation with someone who does not feel any resonation with us. Is this the basis of "I love you, but you don't know I exist?"

Perhaps some people cannot feel resonations. It would reasonable to suggest that people resonate with different strengths and sensitivity. Perhaps others have learned to ignore or avoid resonations. Perhaps some have a yet unexplained, genetically-induced dullness or hypersensitivity.

Resonations are the basis of emotions, and emotion is integral to how we acquire knowledge about a situation and our relationship to it. Coordinating a resonation with objective data is how we federate systems so we can survive. The mirror neurons help decode our ability to understand actions and emotions in others. They may explain the sense that some of us seem more sensitive than others to "vibrations" from those we meet.

Examiners might also ignore certain clues because they are not consistent with their personal goals, experiences or beliefs. Perhaps they want to impress the court with their ability to be tough on crime, or get more work by siding with those who hired them.

My alarm, however, is how often one set of clinicians so frequently find data to support the prosecutor and another set of clinicians so frequently find data to support the defense. Both groups say they do not carry a bias, but the track records prove differently. Formal research breaks down data-gathering and analysis into qualitative and quantitative groups. As I have explained, the qualitative group is the area where one formulates opinions, based on experiences and observations. This is where gut feelings and nuances live.

When two psychologists, using accepted testing scales, can come to different opinions about malingering, it means the "opinion" is based on more than just quantifiable data. The opinion is based too narrowly or too widely on an interpretation of the data. The database does not automatically force a universal result. Totally reliable testing means that only one psychological examination is needed in order to give the courts an accurate finding. Indeed, no new tests and theories would be needed. Many current schemes are diagnostically unreliable. The true nature of science is quite different. Many evaluators ignore that true nature.

In science, we aim for a picture of nature as it really is, unencumbered by any philosophical or theological prejudice. Some see the search for scientific truth as a search for an unchanging reality behind the ever-changing spectacle we observe with our senses. The ultimate prize in that search would be to grasp a law of nature—a part of a transcendent reality that governs all change, but itself never changes.

The idea of eternally true laws of nature is a beautiful vision, but is it really an escape from philosophy and theology? For, as philosophers have argued, we can test the predictions of a law of nature to see if they are verified or contradicted, but we can never prove a law must always be true. So, if we believe a law of nature is eternally true, we are believing in something that logic and evidence cannot establish.

Of course, laws of nature are very useful, and we have been able to discover good candidates for them. But to believe the law is useful and reliable is not the same thing as to believe it is eternally true. We could just as easily believe there is nothing but an infinite succession of approximate laws. Or that laws are generalizations about nature that are not unchanging, but change so slowly that until now we have imagined them as eternal.

As a result, in the past three decades, the attention of physicists has shifted from seeking to know the laws of nature to a new question: why are these laws? Why do these laws, and not others, exist in our universe?[60]

Differing scientific opinions grow into scientific quagmires once a judge makes the final decision. Flawed and inexact science cause the quagmires.

As good as many judges may be, the final clinical decision ought to be made by a panel of mental health experts who would, in turn, deliver their report to the judge. The panel members would be the same people who actually performed the examinations. This way the experts will be forced to reveal their different approaches and 'fess up to their own biases, experiences and differences' in front of colleagues. These differences ought to nullify each other.

When a uniquely specialized or additional expert is needed, the committee will ask for two such professionals to examine the patient and meet with the full committee in order to arrive at a single recommendation. Individual parties can suggest which expert to use, but there can be only one report to the court.

That final recommendation must include a discussion as to why there are differences and how they were resolved. If no consensus can be produced, then the courts should be told that there is insufficient scientific evidence to clearly support its use as a factor in the case.

An attorney could request an expert witness to do an examination outside of the panel's knowledge. The individual attorney would pay for this, or may ask the court to pay for it for indigent clients. However, such information could not, in and of itself, be introduced as a factor in the court's final decision. That data could be the basis of a request that a panel be convened. That original report would then become part of the panel's database, and the expert preparing the report would be part of the panel.

This panel would take the mental health diagnosing aspect of a case away from the judge. The judge would then focus on legal issues only. It would also shrink the lucrative expert witness business as it is now structured.

I imagine such a system will not be well accepted by many mental health professionals who make a good living as expert witnesses. It puts their opinions in an arena where they are being challenged by a peer, not a lawyer with pre-set questions. It also places the entire process of mental health diagnosing under a degree of scrutiny that some mental health professionals may personally find treacherous.

The other mechanism to reduce differences in results would be to establish a national accreditation organization. Every couple of years those who wish to offer opinions to the court must go through a course or refresher course to deal with these issues.

The reason is quite simple. Merely having a professional degree does not equate with being a good diagnostician. We all know that some doctors are better than others. And not all people who make decisions are able to resist their own biases.

Carl Sagan felt that people see their God as "their God" and they want Him to stay that way. This speaks to our human nature—when science cannot be sure of something, then something else will be used to make sense of it. Often that "something else" is a philosophy or religion. "True believers" are convinced their religion is more perfect and better armed to explain human behaviors than is science. The scientist will argue that words like soul or spirit, or "that's his make-up," are just words or phrases for that which cannot yet be explained. Believers allow the word "soul" to carry much more authority than a scientist will give it. A pure scientist would probably not use the word "soul."

Most scientists hold personal convictions that are hybrids of religion, science and evolution.

Einstein himself is quoted as saying: [61]

We are in the position of a little child entering a huge library filled with books in many different languages. The child knows someone must have written those books. It does not know how. The child dimly suspects a mysterious order in the arrangement of the books but doesn't know what it is...

The most beautiful and most profound experience is the sensation of the mystical. It is the sower of all true science. He to whom this emotion is a stranger, who can no longer wonder and stand rapt in awe, is as good as dead. To know that what is impenetrable to us really exists, manifesting itself as the highest wisdom and the most radiant beauty which our dull faculties can comprehend only in their primitive forms - this knowledge, this feeling is at the center of true religiousness.

The brain is a highly-evolved computer designed to solve the engineering problems of taking the body through life. Religion is ultimately a choice but science is not. In the end, two scientists who see the same patient ought to arrive at the same conclusion. That is not necessarily so if two people of different religions are given the same data set. Science is a matter of reporting, religion is a matter of interpreting. Religion is qualitative and science is quantitative. When we need a decision that science cannot provide, we turn to own databanks of beliefs and experiences for the answer. That databank feeds the brain and the brain's software processes until a decision is produced. This progression is exceedingly vulnerable to biases.

Religion should not be desecrated or devalued. It meets many vital human needs. Religion gives answers to loneliness and suffering, and it offers a magical draw that life has meaning behind our earthly and often painful existences. It does nourish a grandiosity of sorts, that, despite what we experience on earth, we are unique and important to a larger universe. That comfort will be the reward if we are good while on earth. Because of this it is the ultimate motivator. It also serves to administer our moral social order.

But religion is also limiting. Many religious standards are human products that have evolved into mechanisms to offer additional social or safety controls, or to preserve a lifestyle. Many challenge those constructs, seeing them as ruses and illusions that do, indeed, provide emotional comfort, but they keep the door closed to the grander schemes of the cosmos and our minds. The pure scientist could classify religion as malingered safety.

The ideal goal for science and religion would be if we could retire the phase, "More than a hunch, and less than a certainty."[62] That retirement is quite far in the future and it cleverly captures the state of affairs in the science and religion on how to detect truth or lying.

Science is ever-changing. To celebrate that, this chapter will end with a return to a discussion of mirror neurons. This is a rapidly evolving field and new information to support or reject the concepts may have not existed when this summary was prepared.

Brain cells that react the same, whether or not an act was done by us, or if we watched someone else do the act, are called mirror neurons. They appear to be the cells that give us the sense of empathy. The Italian researcher, Rizzolatti, observed the same neural patterns when the monkeys grabbed an object or if they just watched another monkey grab the same object. The activity occurred in the prefrontal cortex area known as F5. The "watching" monkey was mirroring the action of the "doing" monkey, almost as if he was saying "Oh, I understand that…I know what that is like…" These same cells have been discovered in humans, and this may be one of the ways in which people understand each other. [63,64]

The first human study of mirror neurons was done in 1995.[65] Though it is harder to identify mirror neuron groups in humans, the concept might fit and explain the origin of the claimed differences in fMRI and other studies to detect lying. Perhaps the psychopathic or the malingering lack normal mirror neuron functioning; this may explain why they feel no empathy with those with whom they are interacting. If they both lacked the neuronal circuitry to respond to the normal clues of social interactions and suffered from psychologically traumatic events, then the ability to empathize is impaired on many dimensions. A mirror neuron requires some personal past experience to lean on. Not having properly functioning mirror neurons converts the world into a wholly present one—no past or future. There may be no, or perhaps only a scant, inventory of prior experiences that contribute any color to a decision.

Given that different mental health professionals commonly interview the same person and come away with different impressions, the disparity may be rooted in the mirror neuron functions within either individual. This includes the patient as well. Critically, this involves concepts such as the halo effect, transference and countertransference. An interviewer with high mirror neuron activity may pick up on traces of emotions in the client. These "pick-ups" will signal where and how the questioning ought to proceed.

The common phrase "Been there, done that, felt that, too" could be a mirror neuron response. Prisoners and patients have mentioned to me that one doctor "seemed to understand me and another doctor just asked questions. I told the first doc a whole lot more about me that I thought I would...man, that one lady really understood me—I felt it. The other guy, man, just a bunch of questions…"

Psychological testing ought to be far removed from such subjective influence, but even examiners using the same test panels can produce different conclusion. Why?

Part of the basic human experience is that we are *not* alienated from the actions, emotions and sensations of others. We are *attuned to the intentional relations of others.* Through an intentional attunement, "the others in our world" are not just different or abstract representational systems; they become *persons*— like us. This produces friendships and trust. It is why we enjoy love songs and cry at sad stories. It is the basis of our literature, our arts and our entertainment.

But there are some who like to keep a boundary between "us" and "them." We invite people into our "us" circle, and when we meet someone who has committed a crime, our moral sense may assign them to the "them" corral. Yet if we look closely at their lives, as often happens in movies and books, we learn that yes, the crime existed, but it was also committed by a real person with many of the same pressures and hopes and loves and losses as ourselves. That phrase, "There, but for the grace of God," rings true.

I have often wondered if those who are more inclined to find malingering are those whose mirror neurons are less active. They remain comfortable not letting the criminal paint the full picture of his life.

"*That new doc, I don't know, he let me feel him. I mean, he had this thing, kinda energy, and I was comfortable with him. That's what they call charisma, right? That first doc, whoa, kinda cold. Like he and I would never have a beer and a laugh. I wanted to tell that second guy not to be so serious... I wondered what his girlfriend was like.*"

CHAPTER EIGHT

The Biology and Biological-Based Detection of Deceit and Malingering

The mode in which the inevitable comes
to pass is effort.
~Oliver Wendell Holmes~

The white-matter volume and connectivity of the human pre-frontal cortex is one of the anatomic variables that separates humans from apes. The pre-frontal cortex maintains a high degree of interaction with numerous other areas of the brain, and if the reader's curiosity is so inclined, a textbook of neuropsychiatry can provide details that are outside the discussion of this book. Most of this book relates to the rather unswerving issues of human nature. This chapter reviews the ever evolving human interface with technology.

It is important to recognize that the dorsolateral (*dorsal* means towards the back, and *lateral* means to the sides) of the prefrontal cortex is associated with decision-making. This "towards the back and to the sides" brain area plays a central role in the temporal organization of behavior. It heavily influences voluntary actions— both in motor movements as well as speech and reasoning. When someone is expected to form and understand how to arrive at a deliberate action, the process takes place in the dorsolateral aspects of the prefrontal cortex. In cooperation with other areas of the brain that constantly provide input, the dorsolateral prefrontal cortex gives a retrospective function of short term memory and a prospective function in preparation for action. These two functions basically reconcile the past with the future. It keeps the actions in a logical order and towards a specific goal. When the dorsolateral prefrontal cortex is not working properly, a disorder can manifest itself with problems of attention, memory, speech, behavior and planning. We are interested in the last problem, planning, although memory and attention problems can influence the ability to properly plan.

Patients with this problem are unable to plan in an organized fashion. They have problems keeping things in mind and executing their plans in an organized manner. Observers of impaired people will say they act irrationally. They may also have problems departing from daily routines and cannot work with novel trends or ideas. There is a dysfunction in the ability to represent and prepare for future action.

Several diagnostic considerations need to be explored if a person has problems planning for the future. The first step is to do a thorough medical and neurological evaluation, including neuropsychological tests. If this finds no explanation, then malingering is possible. A simple check with family or others might give information about other illnesses, injuries, birth abnormalities or any other historical factors—physical or psychological—that will better explain the malingering. Obtaining such data is essential.

It would be ideal to have objective testing instruments to detect malingering. Merely detecting a deception may be adequate for legal issues, but mental health diagnoses demand a motivation for the deception.

These are some new machines and concepts to detect lying. The essential theory behind these instruments is that people cannot alter some basic physiologic process. Once it was felt that a brain wave, known as P300, was always involuntary. This is now known not to be the case, which means that these instruments can be tricked if someone knows how to do it.

Psychopaths show a lack of normal response to fear. They do not anticipate punishment and so have physiologically deficient autonomic activity when faced with what a normal person would experience as fear. For the non-psychopath, this fear comes from experience-induced conditioned discomfort or punishment. Considerable research has been done to identify the brain circuits that gather and maintain conditioned fear. Lesions in the orbitofrontal circuits can lead to "acquired sociopathy." This is demonstrated in socially inadequate choices and irresponsible behavior.[66, 67]

Psychopaths have also been described as emotionally-detached individuals. They do not empathize with the feelings their actions produce in others. A psychopath feels no need to be believed, unlike most people who lie or malinger. Psychopathic malingering is clearly cold and offensive malingering, quite like a deliberate political scam. The offensive malingerers do so to maintain their own power and comfort. Fear is not a motivator, other than the fear of being put out.

Defensive malingers, if caught, feel fear. Offensive malingers feel annoyance when caught. Defensive malingers may pretend to be tougher or stronger than they actually are. They portray an offensive malingering style, but when caught, they feel fear. Very little will induce fear in a psychopathic malinger, and it may be because their neuronal circuitry does not process fear.[68] The tests described may help identify the process of fabrication, but they do little to identify the motivation.

Machine detectors of lying, deceit or malingering involves a technology that is changing so rapidly that it cannot be summarized in a truly up-to-date form. The progress should be monitored with reviews of the legal and medical literatures.

The Polygraph

In 1915, psychologist William Marston invented the polygraph, commonly called the lie detector. This device measures pulse, breathing, perspiration and blood pressure as the person is asked a series of questions with yes or no answers. The theory is that these measures change when a person lies. The polygraph's credibility has been seriously challenged, and in 2003, the National Academy of Sciences reported that little scientific evidence exists to support the trustworthiness of the polygraph.[69] Nonetheless, it is still often used, but most courts will not admit its findings into evidence.

Brain Fingerprinting

Lawrence Farwell measures the brain's burst of activity when the person recognizes something.[70] It is not yet a reliable tool, and Farwell has not shared his data and devices so they can be tested by others. The core concept has some attractions. It is a measure of whether or not some bit of data is in the brain. Based on event-related potentials (ERP), brain fingerprinting looks at the brain's electrical activity in response to a particular stimulus. One bit of the brain's electrical activity is known as the P300, or P3. It is a burst of activity about 300 milliseconds after exposure to a stimulus that has a meaning to the subject. In forensic work, the subject is asked about some detail of the crime that only someone at the crime would know, such as "the victim fell on the green couch…" If the subject knows this, it will have meaning, and the P300 will be evoked.

P300 was thought to be beyond a person's voluntary control, but a 2004 study found that two-thirds of the test subjects could produce P300 waves in situations that should not have been able to produce the P300 waves.[71]

Eye Tracking

Eye tracking is based on the observation that our eyes involuntarily spend less time—a difference in milliseconds—scanning familiar objects than unfamiliar ones. This is another check for concealed knowledge. A criminal's eye ought to spend less time looking at the crime scene than at a picture of a race car.

Infrared Face Scans

Capillaries in the face exhibit small changes in blood flow when the person is under stress. But blood flow changes occur from a long list of triggers, from shyness-based blushing, other causes of anxiety, individual skin and vascular differences, to environmental temperature changes as well. Will the anxious airplane passenger, running late and out of breath, be able to give a normal scan?

And what about the seasoned poker player whose face can be stone cold and unexpressive—could he fool the machine?

fMRI (functional MRI)

In September 2005, the well-respected magazine, *Nature*, published the headline "brain imaging ready to detect terrorists, say neuroscientists."[72]

How wonderful this would be from a national security perspective. Using fMRI techniques, the scientists believe their test is ready for routine use, but many people doubt that the techniques are mature and reliable enough. The attraction of fMRI is based on the belief that subjects cannot hide their deceit. This was the same claim that proponents of the polygraph used for many years until it was disproved.

fMRI, or functional MRI, is based on a brain chemical and electrical changes after events. These events vary with disease and activity. fMRI is different from conventional MRI in that it detects changes in the blood oxygen level-dependant (BOLD) that follow when the there is a change in neuronal activity.[73] A stimulus or task will produce this. Higher levels of BOLD change reflect more neuronal activity. In effect, there are changes, usually decreases, in the amount of free oxygen in the blood, and this is the product of metabolic activity. When the oxygen that is normally bound to hemoglobin is used, the blood is then considered deoxygenated. Deoxygenated blood has a different fMRI signal than does oxygenated blood.

The feeling is that there is a localized brain reaction that correlates to lying, and this reaction cannot be willfully modified. fMRI can measure this brain reaction. During a deception, different brain areas were active when compared to truth telling activities. The following lists are derived from Mohamed:[74]

Areas of the brain active during lying:

Left medial frontal lobe, left inferior frontal lobe, right hippocampus (temporal lobe), right middle temporal gyrus (temporal lobe), left lingual gyrus (occipital lobe), anterior cingulate, right fusisform gyrus, right sublobar insula.

Areas of the brain active during truth telling:

Left subcallosal gyrus (frontal lobe), lentiform nucleus (frontal lobe), left inferior temporal gyrus (temporal lobe)

From the above, it does seem that a lot more effort and energy goes into lying than into telling the truth.

Mohamed also states that, "It is likely that a subject cannot mask functional MRI imaging brain activity." But this may not be so. Birbaumer presented a poster in October 2006 which speaks to the contrary.[75] He showed volunteers a thermometer-like presentation of their insula activity. They were able to control their emotional responses in much the same manner as biofeedback is used to control pain or other emotional events. Healthy people were trained to self-regulate their BOLD response in specific parts of the brain. After some practice, the volunteers could their change reactions to upsetting or non-upsetting images. Birbaumer and Sitaram then performed the same experiment with prison inmates who were classified as being psychopaths. The criminals, who lacked any BOLD response in their fear circuits, also successfully underwent the operant conditioning. The result demonstrated that voluntary control of brain function was possible—even in psychopaths. The psychopath, in effect, obtained more of a normal insula activity.

fMRI may eventually be useful as a detector of lying, but Birhaumer's poster demands that we be very cautious about how fMRI is used. Much more time and work is needed to see if the fMRI approach becomes trustworthy, or if it will eventually be discredited and fall to the side as did the polygraph.

Birhaumer's work poses another chilling question. Apparently psychopaths can be taught to change their emotional reactions to situations. In 2005, Birbaumer reported that psychopaths have a neuronally-based processing flaw that makes them lack any anticipation of aversive or painful events.[76] Their nervous systems seem to lack the autonomic response to threats. They also seem to lack the ability to anticipate harm from indications of danger. In short, the usual stimulus of an aversive event does not condition them to respond with fear when a similar event reappears. The Birhaumer poster seems to suggest that they can at least be re-conditioned enough that their BOLD signals change.

Many of us fear the consequences of lying, so we do not engage in it. We grow up feeling that danger will follow some behaviors. Biological events may predispose to abnormal behaviors, but at this stage of scientific knowledge, and assuming no florid disease state, at best they only increase a sensitivity to events. The bulk of our approaches to life rest on our psychological experiences. Saddam Hussein's sons in Iraq murdered randomly and apparently with no remorse. No one in their country would or could punish them for it. But they did not kill in other countries, so they did have a sense of fear and consequence. If those sons suffered an insula-related event (or even from other parts of the brain), it ought to be active anywhere in the world.

It is commonly assumed that the psychopath has no hesitancy about lying. But lying is not an automatic outgrowth of psychopathy—it has been long assumed that lying would produce fear in the non-psychopathic liar because they fear being caught. If psychopathy is defined, at least in part, by decreased fMRI activity, then lying is psychopathy. Lying in the above fMRI study was done intentionally, so sham lying engages certain brain circuits but this lying stems from a different motivation and history. Is that difference sufficient to rank as valid lying since there is not the typical self-serving background of emotions and motivations?

There has been a common belief that psychopathy is very difficult to remove. Perhaps Birhaumer's work will provide data on how to alter a fear reaction, but will it alter the willful choices that a psychopath makes in life? Some people may not fear a consequence, while others may not care about it. One response may be the BOLD-measurable insula activity that induces fear. Not having fear may enable a psychopathic personality to flourish. But could a psychopathic personality still develop, even with insula-generated fear? Many psychopaths are very narcissistic, and many narcissists are very fearful. They arrange their lives in ways that reduce their exposure to the fears.

The unknowns are intriguing, and it will be so fascinating to watch new data go through the revealing debates.

CHAPTER NINE

Brief Endnotes

Ah, but a man's reach should exceed his grasp
~Browning~

My own psychoanalysis left me with a legacy to top off any project with some free association. Doing so tugs on the newly sewn garment—the stitches tighten and the shape takes hold. So—

What do we really know about a lie? A lie is an intent. It is no more than a masqueraded form of some truth. Peeling back the camouflage that a lie desperately wants to be identified as truth reveals the subterranean dodge and game.

Those who disagree about the presence or not of malingering must be judging the same data through different biases, otherwise there would not be any substantive differences. Perhaps they invite or filter inputs which reduce the persuasions of the qualitative data used in the quantitative analysis. Such affiliations produce different *gestalts*. To homogenize the trustworthiness of opinions, each observer should test his own biases. A gestalt bias is assessed by the gestalt switch, during which the examiner or judge revisits the evaluation using another set of personal, political, and professional gestalts. The perception that something is inaccurate simply because the other side has offered it is referred to as a "reactive devaluation." Many people tend to ignore that personal selections do affect their judgment. This potential bias in evaluating behaviors has been called the "fundamental attribution error."

Many consider a lie as the mask of a coward. The liar lacks the courage to be truthful. Being honest carries as many ramifications as being dishonest, and the coward *qua* liar is afraid of some penalty. The coward is intentionally put before the *qua*.

Apparently fearing the *truth ramification* can be worse than the fear of a *lie ramification*. How the person responds to being caught reflects the motivation for the lie. We must ask if those who lie do so because they are not brave enough or feel safe enough to be honest, or if they lie because they are cocky and indifferent to anything outside of their own needs. A lie brings cold light to a situation. Honesty brings the sun's warmth. Interestingly, the Sanskrit word for courage is *saurya*, which has its roots in the Sanskrit word for sun.

Where is the emotional and spiritual center of those who malinger? Why can they not just surrender to their fears and problems and ask, straight out, for help? What arrogance or distasteful experience persuaded them to choose tactics which can only cause profound battles and disharmony? One difference between the offensive and the defensive malingerer is that the offensive malingerer often has an inner stillness and joy about his malingering. The defensive malingerer is not at peace.

A lie is disrespectful. It exploits the listener. When an honest speaker communicates towards others, we often feel an empathy for their position or assignment. To have such empathy lives in the phrase "to have a heart." Being honest with listeners is to respect them. It takes courage to be honest. And the word courage itself comes from the French, *coeur*, meaning heart. To be honest and courageous is therefore to have a heart and be charitable or respectful to those with whom we interact.

A lie is truth twisted. It is incapable of being shared. Those who lie want those who are lied to not to see it is a lie. That is the operational focus. But those to whom the lie is directed have to test the lie, and if it does not fit the common human experience, the lie cannot be accepted as truth. The liar has a grandiosity that he, unlike all others, can invent a lie so compelling and so unique that common human experience cannot correctly evaluate it. As such, it is expected to be accepted.

An odd deception must exist in the liar's mind. Lying, or malingering, requires that the malingerer holds two contradictory beliefs in his mind simultaneously; he has to accept both ideas as real.

A lie is a hidden truth. The cruelest lie is holding a truth in silence. Untimely truths told with bad intent may do as much harm as a lie—such truths indeed need unveiling, but with some savvy and diplomacy so as not to be delivered as bombs or in the midst of revenge.

Truth exists; only lies are invented. Truth is not manmade and withstands any scrutiny. The truth of a lie is exposed under scrutiny.

We all need to survive. We survive with only the tools at our disposal, and we compete to bring energy into our lives to feed and preserve our bodies and our egos.

One of the staple duties is clear-cut. We must unfold the folded lie. Therein will appear the hidden truth. Just as a miserly baker wraps extra layers of less expensive pastry dough to hide his shortened measure of sweet filling, so too does an experienced child unfold the pastry to see if he has received a fair portion of the tasty treat. We must be that child.

REFERENCES

1. Heterdox means unconventional or unorthodox. Copernicus's "the sun is the center of our solar system" theory was initially heterodoxy. Warburton's "Orthodoxy...is my doxy - heterodoxy is another man's doxy," captures the observation that people often presume their own ideas as accurate while others' are wide of the mark. Antonyms, orthodox and heterodox stem from the Greek doxa, which means "opinion," and Heterodox adds doxa plus heter, "other" or "different." "Orthodoxy" joins "doxa" with orth-, to mean "correct" or "straight."

2   "Calumny" is the act of uttering false charges or misrepresentations maliciously calculated to harm another's reputation. Its origin is from the Latin *calvi*, meaning "to deceive." Conceivably a biased or less than scientifically scrupulous examiner could color a reputation by even suggesting the presence of a malingering. The burden of undoing this "suggestion of malingering" can be formidable.

3   Linebarger, Paul Myron Anthony. 1954. Psychological Warfare, 1954, Combat Forces Press, Washington (p. 39)

4   *malinger*. Dictionary.com. Unabridged (v 1.0.1). Random House, Inc. http://dictionary.reference.com/browse/malinger (accessed: December 06, 2006).

5   Resnick, P.J.: Malingering of posttraumatic stress disorders. In Resnick, R., ed: Clinical Assessment of Malingering and Deception. 2nd ed. New York: Guilford Press;1997:130–152

6   Rogers, R. Introduction. In: Rogers, R, ed. Clinical Assessment of Malingering and Deception 2nd ed. New York. Guilford Press; 1997: 1–19

7   This immediately triggers the philosophical debate on how to distinguish between "lying" and the oft and well-rationalized relative to lying known as "fudging." There is no difference—they are both falsifications.

8   Dalby, J.F.: The Case of Daniel McNaughton: Let's Get The Story Straight. American Journal of Forensic Psychiatry. 2006; 27(4): 17–31

9   Pierre, J.M., Wirshing, D.A., Witshing, W.C.: Iatrogenic Malingering. Psychiatric Services. Feb. 2003 (54–2); 253–254

10 Kasdan, M.L.: Malingering by proxy: a form of pediatric falsification (case report). Journal of Development and Behavioral Pediatrics. 2003; August 24 (4):276–8

11 Elwyn, T.S., Ahmed, I.: Factitious Disorder. April 2006 www.emedicine.com/med/topic3125.htm   Accessed November 17, 2006

12 Thorndike, E.L.: A Constant Error on Psychological Rating. Journal of Applied Psychology. 1920 (4)25–29

13 http://pespmc1.vub.ac.be/:/ASC/HAWTHO_EFFEC.html, assessed December 6, 2006

14 Scand, J. Work Environ Health. 2006 Oct;32(5):402–12

15 Adelman, R.M., Howard A. Expert testimony on malingering: The admissibility of clinical procedures for the detection of deception. Behavioral Sciences and the Law. 1984:2;5–19

16 The word *execrate* stems from the Latin verb *exsecrari*, which means to put under a curse. More contemporary use of this word suggests a declaration that something is evil, detestable, or needs to be denounced. The word itself is a combination of components which means "not sacred," which is a character denigration.

17 Kraepelin, E.: Die Erscheinungsformen des Irreseins {translated by H. Marshall as: Patterns of mental disorder}. In: Hirsch, S.R., Shepherd, M., eds. Themes and Variations in European Psychiatry. Bristol, England: Wright; 1974:7–30. Z Gesamte Neurol Psychiat. 1920:62:1–29

18 Hume, D.: "Of Miracles" An Enquiry Concerning Human Understanding. Beuachamp TL, ed., Oxford: Oxford University Press, 1999

19 Is it not interesting that the word "win" is applied to a verdict? One should not need to win a verdict of truth and scientific fact. Patients do not "win" their diagnoses.

20 To *vilify* is a strong deprecatory term. It regards the person as worthless or of little value. The term itself comes from Latin *vilis* for vile or worthless. "Vilipend" also includes the verb *pendere*, which means to weigh, and as such, to *vilipend* is to find someone not worth considering.

21 Rosenberg, Sarah. "Face." *Beyond Intractability*. Eds. Guy Burgess and Heidi Burgess. Conflict Research Consortium, University of Colorado, Boulder. Posted: February 2004 http://www.beyondintractability.org/essay/face/.

22 Davidson, R.J.: Prolegomenon to the structure of emotion: gleanings from neuropsychology. Cognition and Emotion. 1992;6:245–268

23 Serin, R. Psychopathy and violence in criminals. Journal of Interpersonal Violence. 1991:6:423-431

24 "Fictitious," from Latin *ficticius*, means "artificial" or "feigned." It was used as an antonym for "natural." *Ficticius* , also from the Latin *fingere*, "to shape, form, or devise." "Fictitious" is typically applied to imaginative creations or feigned emotions.

25 Factitious is used to suggest something synthetic, forced, simulated or counterfeit. Fictitious has a flavor of being fanciful, unreal, illusory or dishonest. The overlaps are obvious.

26 Kaplan, H., Sadock, B.: Synopsis of Psychiatry. Eighth Edition. Williams and Wilkins, 1988, pg 861

27 Hutchinson, G.L.: Disorders of Simulation: Malingering, Factitious Disorders and Compensation Neurosis. Madison, Conn. Psychological Press 2001.

28 Burber, M, Kaufman W. I and Thou. New York. Macmillan, 1970 (Original in 1923)

29 Clark, C.: Sociopathy, malingering, and defensiveness, in Clinical Assessment of Malingering and Deception. 2en Ed. Edited by Rogers, R. New York, Guilford, 1997

30   Poythress, N.G., Edens, J.F., Watkins, M.M.: The relationship between psychopathic personality features and malingering symptoms of major mental illness. Law and Human Behavior. 25;567–582, 2001

31   Richards, L.: Extract from Black Propaganda — Clandestine Psychological Warfare of WWII. www.psywar.org. Accessed January 24, 2007

32   American Psychiatric Association: Diagnostic and Statistical Manual of Mental Disorders. Fourth Ed, Text Revision, Washington DC; American Psychiatric Association, 2000

33   Daghestani, A.N., Dinwiddle, S.H., Hardy, D.W.: Antisocial Personality Disorders in and out of correctional and forensic settings. Psychiatric Annuals. 2001;31(7):441–446

34   Goodwin, R.D., Hamilton, S.P.: Lifetime co-morbidity of antisocial personality disorder and anxiety disorders among adults in the community. Psychiatry Research. 2003 Feb 15; 117(2):159-66

35   Geiger, B.: Crime, Prostitution, Drugs and Malingered Insanity. International Journal of Offender Therapy and Comparative Criminology. 2006;50(5): 582–594

36   Deuteronomy is from late Latin *deuteronomium* and from Greek *deuteronomion*, meaning a second law (*deuteros*, second + *nomos*, law). The name, Deuteronomy, comes from the name given to the book by both the Septuagint and the Vulgate (Deuteronomium). The Septuagint mistranslated the Hebrew as a second-giving of the law. However, it is not inappropriate because Deuteronomy includes both new material and a number of the laws found in Exodus

37   Meloy, J.R.: Antisocial Personality Disorder. In: Gabbard, G., ed. Treatments of Psychiatric Disorders. Vol 2. Washington DC. American Psychiatric Press. 1995:2273–2290

38   Meloy, J.R.: The Psychology of Wickedness: Psychopathy and Sadism. Psychiatric Annals. 1997,27:9 (September); 630–633

39   Kim-Cohen, J., Caspi, A., Taylor, A., et al: MAOA, maltreatment and gene-environment predicting children's mental health: new

evidence and a meta-analysis. Molecular Psychiatry. 2006, 11: 903–913

40   Jacob, C.P., Muller, J., Schmidt, M.: Cluster B Personality Disorders are Associated with Allelic Variation of Monoamine Oxidase A Activity. Neuropsychopharmacology. 2005, 30:1711–1718

41   Adler, M.: The World of the Talmud. B'nai B'rith Hillel Foundations, Inc. Philadelphia, 1958, p 80

42   Caspi, A., McClay, J., Moffitt, T.E. et al. (2002) Role of genotype in the cycle of violence in maltreated children. Science 297(5582): 851–854

43   Olds, D., Henderson, C.R. Jr., Cole, R. et al. (1998). Long term effects of nurse home visitation on children's criminal and antisocial behavior: 15 year follow-up of a randomized control trial. JAMA 280(14):1238–1244

44   Donegan, N.H., Sanislow, C.A., Blumberg, H.P. et al. (2003) Amygdala hyperactivity in borderline personality disorder: implication for emotional dysregulation. Biol Psychiatry 54(11):1284–1293

45   First Samuel 21:14

46   Preuss, J.: Biblical and Talmudic Medicine. Rosner, F., translator and editor, Jason Aronson Inc, New Jersey and London, 1993; 311–321

47   Burton R.: Anatomy of Melancholy. New York. New York Review of Books 2001

48   Synedeham T.: Processes Integri. In Clending L.: Source Book of Medical History. New York. Courier Dover Publications, 1960

49   Hart, B.: The Psychology of Insanity (3rd Ed.), Cambridge University Press, 1912

50   Münsterberg, H.: On The Witness Stand. Essays on Psychology and Crime. Doubleday, Page and Co., New York, 1913

51   Klein, I.: Response Expectancy as a determinant of experience and behavior. Am Psychol 40:1985, 1189–1202

52   American Psychological Association (2002). Ethical principles of psychologists and code of conduct. Am Psychol 57:1060–1073. Available: www.apa.org/ethics

53   The answer is obvious. She is beautiful to someone. We must look at the beauty of her soul.

54   Bok, S.: Lying: Moral Choice in Public and Private Life. New York, Vintage Books 1999

55   www.wordorigins.org/index.php/site/comments/merriam_websters_word_of_the_year, accessed October 5, 2008

56   One aspect of good psychiatric training is that students needed to undergo their own psychotherapy. This helps them identify their own biases and countertransferences which, in turn, may influence how they formulate diagnoses in their patients.

57   Frye v. United States, 293 F. 1013 (D.C. Cir. 1923)

58   Bendectin was used to control nausea during pregnancy. The medication was voluntarily withdrawn from the market in the 1983.

59   Daubert v. Merrell Dow Pharmaceuticals, Inc., 509 U.S. 579 (1993),

60   Smolin L. Never Say Always. New Scientist 23 September 2006: 31–35.

61   Einstein A: The Merging of Spirit and Science. http://www.spaceandmotion.com/Theology-Albert-Einstein.htm, accessed October 19, 2008

62   Barash, D.P. (2006). More than a hunch, and less than a certainty. A review of Douglas W. Mock, More Than Kin and Less Than Kind: The Evolution of Family Conflict. Harvard University Press, Cambridge, MA, 2006. Evolutionary Psychology, 4, 459–461.

63   Di Pellegrino, G., Fadiga L., Fogassi, L., Gallose, V., Rizzolatti G: Understanding motor events: a neurophysiological study Exp Brain Res. 1992; 91(1):176–180

64   Gallose, V., Fogassi, L., Fadiga, L., Rizzolatti, G.: Action recognition in the pre-motor cortex. Brain 1996;119(2);593–609

65   Rizzolatti, G., Fadiga, L.: Motor facilitation during action observation: a magnetic stimulation study. J Neurophysiology. 1995 Jun;73(6):2608–11

66 Damasio, A.R.: A neural basis for sociopathy. Arch Gen Psychiatry. 2000;57:128–129

67 Anderson, S.W., Bechara, A., Damasio, H., et al: Impairment of social and moral behavior related to early damage in human prefrontal cortex. Nat Neurosci 1999;2:1032–1037

68 Birbaumer, N., Veit, R., Lotzes, M.: Deficient Fear Conditioning in Psychopathy. Arch Gen Psychiatry 2005;62:799–805

69 National Research Council. The Polygraph and Lie Detection. National Academies Press, Washington DC, 2003

70 Farwell, L.A., Donchin, E.: The Truth Will Out: interrogative polygraphy ("lie detection") with event-related brain potentials. Psychophysiology. 1991; Aug (28)5; 531–547

71 Rosenfeld, J.P., Soskins, M., Bosh, G., Ryan, A.: Simple, effective countermeasures to P300-based tests of detection of concealed information Psychophysiology 2004; Mar (41)2: 205–219

72 Wild, J.: Brain Imaging ready to detect terrorists, say neuroscientists. Nature 2005; Sept 437:22;457

73 Gore, J.: Principles and practice of functional MRI of the human brain. J Clin Investigation 2003: Jul (12)1; 4–9

74 Mohamed, F,. Faro, S., Gorom, N., et al: Brain Mapping of Deception and Truth Telling about an Ecologically Valid Situation. Radiology. 238(2): Feb 2006;679 688

75 Birbaumer, N., Sitaram, R.: BCI-regulation of neuronal substrates of emotions. Presented as a poster at the Society for Neuroscience meeting, October 2006.

76 Birhaumer, N., Veit, R., Lotze, M.: Deficient fear conditioning in psychopathy. Arch Gen Psychiatry. 2005; 62:799–805

INDEX

guilt, 9, 26, 27, 39
guilt as moral compass, 26
gut feeling, 74

H

habitual criminality, 45
hallucinations, 10, 51, 65
halo effect, 14, 16, 17, 58, 78
Hamilton, 90
Hamilton and ASPD, 40
hanger (French), 7
Hart, 51, 90
Hart and insanity symptoms, 51
Hawthorne effect in workplace, 17
heterodox, 5, 88
hierarchical malingering, 6, 11, 30
high context cultures, 26
high context societies, 25
Hippocrates, 6, 50
Hirstein, 12
histrionic, 7
histrionic personality disorder, 52
histro -(Latin), 7
honesty, 49, 60
honesty in social contracts, 11
Howard, 17, 88
humiliation and shame, 25
Hutchinson, 37, 89
hypochondriasis, 16, 52
hysteria, 50
hysteria and malingering, 52

I

I don't remember, 5
iatrogenic disorders, 18
iatrogenic malingering, 6, 14

illness and factitious disorder, 36
illness denial, 13
illness genuine, 37
illness hiding, 12
immature brains, 53
immature psychology, 53
impaired people, 80
individualistic societies, 26
infrared face scans, 28, 82
injurious lie, 56
innocuous lie, 56
insanity, 10, 38, 50
insanity not guilty by reason there of, 22
insanity plea, 21
insanity-malingered, 40
insula, 85
insula activity and emotions, 83, 84
insula generated fear, 85
integrity, 44, 59, 60
intent of the act, 21
intentional attunement, 78
Israeli Mizrahi women, 40

J

J.F. Kennedy, 70
jocose lie, 56
Josh Billings, 36, 70
judge, 53, 54, 71, 72, 75, 76, 86
judgment-impaired, 34
judgment-mature, 34
junk science, 20, 62, 71, 72, 75
jury, 20, 72

K

Karl Menninger, 6
keeping clinical objectivity, 16
King David malingered, 49

Q